IN MY HANDS

IN MY HANDS

Compelling Stories from a Surgeon and His
Patients Fighting Cancer

STEVEN A. CURLEY, MD, FACS

CENTER
STREET

New York   Nashville

Copyright © 2018 by Steven A. Curley, MD

Cover design by Edward A. Crawford
Cover photograph by Getty Images
Cover copyright © 2018 by Hachette Book Group, Inc.

Center Street
Hachette Book Group
1290 Avenue of the Americas, New York, NY 10104
centerstreet.com
twitter.com/centerstreet

First Edition: May 2018

Center Street is a division of Hachette Book Group, Inc. The Center Street name and logo are trademarks of Hachette Book Group, Inc.

The publisher is not responsible for websites (or their content) that are not owned by the publisher.

Library of Congress Control Number: 2017963558

ISBN: 978-1-5460-8270-5 (hardcover), 978-1-5460-8269-9 (ebook)

Printed in the United States of America

LSC-C

10 9 8 7 6 5 4 3 2 1

To my wife, Natalie.
Thank-you will never be enough.

CONTENTS

INTRODUCTION

My parents are native New Mexicans. My mother was born in Taos and my father in Albuquerque. They were both born during the Great Depression, a few years before the onset of World War II. That was when the population of humans in New Mexico was only slightly greater than the population of coyotes.

I am the only member of my extended family not born in either New Mexico or Colorado. I was born in the panhandle of Texas, where my father was playing professional, minor-league baseball at the time. At age six weeks, I moved to New Mexico with my parents, so I have no recollection of my time as a Texan. My grandfather, my mother's father, always called me Tex. It was not a term of endearment.

Growing up in New Mexico in the 1960s and '70s was a simple and pleasant experience. My impressions of the world came from movies or television, on the rare times when my brother and I were allowed to watch it, but mostly they came from books. I loved to read, and books were my source of adventure, education, and imagination. I voraciously devoured history and fiction with equal gusto. Reading was the only way I thought I would ever visit places beyond my immediate borders. My teachers were wise enough to recognize that I needed activities to keep me busy—and to prevent me from chatting with my neighbors when I finished my work. So they plied me with books and writing assignments to describe the adventures and historical events I learned about in my readings.

Along with our friends, my brother and I wandered the mesas and arroyos at the base of the Sandia Mountains in Albuquerque. We played baseball, football, basketball, and every make-believe game we could imagine. In retrospect, ours was a rather idyllic existence.

I didn't realize New Mexico was a climatically, culturally, and geographically diverse state until I was in college. I was the first member of my entire family to attend college, much less obtain a university degree. As an undergrad, I decided to apply to medical school. Using my parents' home address, I sent a form letter to more than forty medical schools throughout the United States requesting information about their programs and application processes. Every school except one replied by providing a description of their courses and requirements for admission. The one exception was the University of Oklahoma Health Sciences Center in Oklahoma City. Parenthetically, the panhandle of Oklahoma borders the far northeast corner of New Mexico. Rather than a booklet describing the medical school experience at the University of Oklahoma, I received a personal letter from the dean of the school. He thanked me for my interest in the program but went on to tell me that, regrettably, the University of Oklahoma did not accept applications from foreign students.

Clearly, the dean was geographically challenged. Technically New Mexico and Oklahoma are neighboring states. I shared the letter with several of my friends, including one who was a political science major. We all thought it was very funny, and my friend showed the letter to one of his professors in the Department of Political Science. The professor was a retired United States senator from the state of Oklahoma. We mistakenly thought he would laugh when he read the letter. He did not. He was outraged. He had the dean of the medical school on the phone within minutes and gave him a brief but direct lesson on the geography of the United States. Subsequently, the dean told the professor I should definitely apply to medical school at the University of Oklahoma.

No thanks.

I like stories, whether told by a masterful chronicler of tales or written in a book or magazine. I always enjoy learning new things and exploring new places I can visualize in my imagination. It amazes me that my career as an academic surgical oncologist has allowed me to visit hundreds of places I could only wistfully dream of actually seeing as a boy: the pyramids of Giza, the Colosseum in Rome, the Great Wall of China, dozens of other manmade marvels, and natural wonders and vistas on every continent except Antarctica (it's on the bucket list).

One of the storytellers I admire is Ernie Pyle, a famous World War II news correspondent who, like me, lived in Albuquerque. A Pulitzer Prize–winning journalist, Pyle was known for his accounts of everyday, otherwise-anonymous people and, in wartime, for his extraordinary features on ordinary soldiers. He wrote clean, clear, crisp stories and painted word pictures capable of evoking great emotion. Sadly, Ernie Pyle was killed while embedded with a division of army troops attempting to take Ie Island in April 1945, before the invasion of Okinawa.

I am no Ernie Pyle, but this is a book of stories about some of my real patients and real situations in modern cancer care. I like to tell stories that have inspired me. It's how I encourage patients dealing with the fear and uncertainty that come with a diagnosis of cancer. Not all of the stories have happy endings. But I recognize that patients relate to the harsh realities faced by other people dealing with the same potentially grim outcome. And they can find empathy and comfort in knowing they are not alone. For privacy reasons, I cannot identify patients by name or specific characteristics that would allow them to be recognized, but all the patients and families described in this book are actual people, individuals who have demonstrated remarkable characteristics and virtues that have been a lesson and blessing to me and others involved in their care. For the few chapters in which information is divulged that might identify a specific patient, express written consent to publish the story was obtained from the patient and/or family.

In 1971 President Richard Nixon declared a "war on cancer," which led to Congress's passing the National Cancer Act the same year. If we are at war with cancer, it is by far the longest and most costly conflict in the history of the United States. The list of Americans killed or injured by cancer and our treatments is prodigious. The socioeconomic burden for cancer care in the United States and worldwide is mind-boggling. The impact of a cancer diagnosis on patients, their families, friends, and co-workers is profound and life-altering. The loss of productivity, skills, financial security, and normal lifestyle is staggering. And the emotional burden for patients and their caregivers—whether soon after diagnosis or when death from a progressive and incurable disease becomes inevitable—is incalculable and imponderable.

But ponder we must. The war on cancer continues. Here and there we win minor victories and even occasional major battles. The enemy is still active, however, and the cost in human lives and well-being is unacceptable. These accounts from the front lines represent a small fraction of the patients I have been privileged to care for during my career as a surgical oncologist. I am mindful of the virtues displayed by these common but remarkable people because they are a daily gift granted unconditionally to me. Some of the narratives describe important experiences

about preparedness and what I learned from the occasional seren-
dipitous opportunity.

My goal is to share these gifts from my patients and to honor all
patients, family members, friends, acquaintances, and caregivers
who have been or still are involved in the fight against cancer. I
respect you all.

Fight on!

IN MY HANDS

1

A Fishing Story

"Hope is being able to see that there is light despite all
of the darkness."

Desmond Tutu

*Hope: A feeling of expectation and desire for a certain
thing to happen*

I learn useful life lessons from each patient I meet. Some are positive messages, reminding me of the importance of maintaining
balance between family, work, and leisure activities. But more
frequently I witness examples of the remarkable resilience of the
human spirit when faced with a diagnosis of cancer and the reality and risks of a major surgical procedure. Occasionally patients
and their family members utter sad remarks when they are faced
with a grim prognosis and the emotions associated with onrushing mortality. Their comments invariably involve an inventory
of regrets, including, "I should have spent more time with my
kids," "I wish I had told my father (or mother, brother, sister, child,
or some other person) that I loved them before they died," and

"I have spent my entire life working, I never took time for any-thing else." I wince when I hear openly expressed regret; I recog-nize I am hearing painful and heartfelt truths. Every week I am reminded that I do not want to look back at my life with a long list of regrets, things I'll wish I had done, and what-ifs.

Early in my academic career I was blessed to meet a great teacher in the guise of a patient. He came to my clinic during my first year as an assistant professor of surgery, shortly after I completed a fellowship in surgical oncology. My patient was a sixty-nine-year-old Baptist minister from a small town in Missis-sippi. His medical oncologist referred him to me. The physician called me and said, "I don't think there is anything you can do for him, but he needs to hear that from you because he doesn't believe me." This tall, imposing patient had colon cancer that had metastasized to his liver. The malignant tumor in his colon had been removed the year before I met him, and he had received chemotherapy to treat several large tumors found in his liver. How-ever, the chemotherapy had not worked and the tumors had grown. The medical oncologist told him he would live no more than six months, and because he was an avid fisherman when he was not preaching or helping others in his community, the doctor sug-gested that he go out and enjoy his remaining time by getting in as much fishing as possible.

I learned two invaluable lessons from this patient and his fam-ily. First, never deny or dismiss a patient's hope, even when from a medical perspective the situation seems hopeless and the patient is incurable. Second, quoting the minister directly, "Some doc-tors think of themselves as gods with a small g, but not one of you is God."

When I first walked into the exam room, this man was slouched on the examining table in the standard blue-and-white, open-backed, unflattering hospital gown. He briefly made eye contact with me and then looked down to the floor. In that momentary glance, I saw no sparkle, no life, and no hope in his eyes. He responded to my initial questions with a monotonic and quiet voice. Several times I had to ask him to repeat an answer because his response was so muted. Midway through our first visit, the patient's wife told me he had been very depressed by his diagnosis of untreatable, metastatic colon cancer. She reported—despite his occasional side-long warning glances requesting her silence—that while he was eating well, he was spending most of his time sitting in a chair or lying in bed. And that the active, gregarious man with the quick wit and booming voice that she had married was gone.

After I interviewed and examined the minister, I left the room and reviewed the results of the lab tests and computed tomography (CT) scans we had performed on him. When I returned to the room he was dressed and sitting in a chair next to his wife. I explained to them that I believed it was possible to perform a difficult operation that would remove approximately 80 percent of his liver. The operation would be risky, there was a potential that he would require blood transfusions, and, as a worst-case scenario, the small amount of remaining liver might not be sufficient to perform necessary functions. If I pushed the surgical envelope too far and removed too much normal liver, following the operation he could develop liver failure leading rapidly to his death. I also stated that, assuming he survived the major operation and the recovery period, I could not predict his long-term outcome or survival. I emphasized that even if the operation were successful, it would be possible that the cancer would recur in the remaining liver or in some other organ. I even attempted to raise his spirits a bit by injecting some puerile surgical wordplay when I said, "This operation will leave you with little more than a sliver of liver, but God willing it will be enough!"

At the conclusion of my very direct monologue, he looked up from the floor and once again his eyes met mine. I remember blinking in surprise several times at how different he now appeared. With his eyes bright and twinkling he asked, "Are you saying there is hope?"

I replied that I believed there was hope, albeit small and impossible to measure, but hope nonetheless.

An unforgettable and immediate transformation in his demeanor occurred, and his wife smiled at me as she mouthed the words, "He's back." He reverted instantaneously to what I would come to learn was his former, garrulous self.

The spiritually resuscitated minister sat upright, grasped my right hand with both of his hands, and launched into a memorable diatribe. "Never deny someone hope, Doctor, no matter how hopeless you know the situation to be. Humans need hope, without it there is depression, despair, and death. Why do you think the Jewish defenders at Masada held out against an overwhelming Roman force for so long? Because they had hope and they had faith. Why do people let you cut them open? Hope. Never deny a human being hope, Doctor. Without it we have no humanity; we are only another animal."

He was a forceful and eloquent speaker. With his Mississippi drawl, he could alternatively be plainspoken or pedantic. I discovered he was a well-read and educated man and he loved to display his extensive lexical armamentarium. Not infrequently after our conversations I would seek out a dictionary to learn the meaning of a word or two. I had no difficulty visualizing him preaching from the pulpit in his Baptist church, like a yo-yo dropping his parishioners to the floor with the fear of eternal damnation, and then pulling them back up into his hands with a message of redemption and salvation.

Enthralled, I walked out of the examination room and

scheduled the operation for the next week. I was amazed by the sudden change I had witnessed in this man's posture and overall demeanor. Like many who provide care for people with debilitating medical conditions, I have seen patients lapse into a state of abject despair. Their spiritual demise leads to a rapid downward spiral of their physical condition. These patients fulfill the expectations of medical practitioners who have told them their survival will be a matter of only weeks or a few months. In fact I have seen several patients die much sooner than I would have predicted when darkness and despair overwhelmed them.

I had the minister's "sermon" on my mind throughout his operation. As I expected, the procedure was technically difficult. He was a robust, barrel-chested man and had four large tumors in his liver. All four were in the right lobe of liver, but two of them extended into portions of the left lobe. One also extended down to involve two of the three large veins that drain blood from the liver into the inferior vena cava, the large vein that carries blood back to the heart. To assure that I had completely removed the tumor around these two veins, I took out a portion of the wall of the inferior vena cava and replaced it with a patch from another vein. It was a liver surgery tour de force, and when it was over, the surgical fellow who performed the operation with me and I quietly congratulated each other on a job well done. Nonetheless, I admit to having had my own negative sentiments and a paucity of optimism. I remarked to the surgical fellow that while the operation had been technically challenging and a great lesson in surgical anatomy, I doubted that we had cured this patient. I was concerned that the aggressive cancer would return.

"Never deny someone hope, Doctor." If I ever had a crystal ball to predict the future, I obviously dropped it in the mud a long time ago. I was wrong about the minister. His cancer never returned. He spent only one week in the hospital after his surgery and his

sliver of liver performed and regenerated beautifully. For the first five years I saw him every three to six months with lab tests and CT scans to check for the return of malignant tumors. For the next six years I saw him only for an annual visit. This man survived and enjoyed life for eleven years after being told he had only six months to live. He died at age eighty, as many of us would wish to die, in his sleep from a stroke. He gave his last sermon from the pulpit of his church three days before he died. His cancer never returned to prey upon his mind and hunt down his hope.

After thinking about it, I realize I learned one additional lesson from this patient. He taught me that it was acceptable to express a little clean, righteous anger and then laugh and move on. The minister and I developed a ritual we repeated at each of his visits after passage of the initial six months his medical oncologist gave him. Once I reviewed the results of his tests and CT scans and confirmed that all was well and the cancer had not returned, he would smile and say, "Let's do it!" From the examining room, I would dial the phone number of the medical oncologist in Mississippi. The minister admitted to me he was angry that this doctor had needlessly denied him hope. When the oncologist came on the line, I would hand the phone to the minister, who would identify himself, and then he would say exactly the same words, each time, "Hey, Doc, you want to go fishing?"

As a surgeon, I confess I enjoyed witnessing the precision with which the preacher inserted this verbal blade, deftly turning it to maximize the impact of his statement. When I passed the phone to the minister, he always had an impish, perhaps even devilish, grin on his face. After he asked the doctor if he would care to join him for a fishing expedition, he would hand the phone back to me and a look of serenity would come over him. The ritual was completed when I would take the phone and speak to the doctor in Mississippi. In my first few conversations with the physician, I apologized for my obvious and indecorous breach in professional behavior. But to the credit of this man being regularly taunted by a Baptist minister, who wasn't entirely forgiving, he would tell me that no apology was necessary and he believed he deserved, and benefited from, the brief but poignant verbal reminders. As the years passed, the doctor would be laughing when I put the phone to my ear, telling me that he really enjoyed the calls and his whole office staff looked forward to this annual event.

The doctor in Mississippi told me it was because of the minister that he never answered patients with a diagnosis of advanced cancer about their expected longevity. Instead, he would inform patients and their families he really couldn't make such a prediction. Not only because of marked individual differences in responses to treatment, but because of the immeasurable will to live—even in individuals no longer receiving treatment for their cancer. Together, he and I learned the importance of leaving no stone unturned in treatment: to engage in multidisciplinary management and to consider all options for our patients. Great lessons from a great spiritual teacher taught to a couple of hardheaded doctors.

"Hey, Doc, you want to go fishing?"

2

Heroes Walking among Us

"I learned that courage was not the absence of fear, but the triumph over it. The brave man is not he who does not feel afraid, but he who conquers that fear."

Nelson Mandela

Courage: The ability to do something that frightens one; bravery; strength in the face of pain, fear, or grief

Living among us, usually unbeknownst to us, are people who have experienced war. I am reminded of these men and women every anniversary of V-E Day, May 8. Victory in Europe Day commemorates the unconditional surrender of Germany to the Allies, and the end of World War II in Europe.

My grandfather and two of his brothers fought with the U.S. Army in Europe during the war. One of my great-uncles went ashore in Normandy on D-Day. My grandfather and my other great-uncle soon followed with the waves of Allied troops that arrived in France in the weeks after June 6, 1944. All three saw combat in France and Germany, and all three received commendations and medals, including a Bronze Star for my great-uncle who fought at Bastogne during the Battle of the Bulge.

None of these men ever talked much about their time in Europe in World War II. However, shortly before he died, one of my great-uncles told me, "I saw things you can't imagine, and memories that I can't wash away." He then told me he'd been in the contingent of U.S. soldiers that liberated prisoners from Buchenwald in April 1945. When I looked at pictures in books of the emaciated Jewish prisoners, I couldn't believe what I saw, and I knew he couldn't either.

During my rotations at the Veterans Administration Hospital as a general-surgery resident I was honored to care for many veterans of World War II, Korea, and Vietnam. I listened intently to their stories, recognizing the opportunity to learn history from actual participants. While some, like my grandfather and great-uncles, did not talk much about their involvement, others told remarkable stories of harrowing survival and astonishing experiences. In my career as a surgical oncologist I have continued to learn from the firsthand stories told by veterans and their families. I always feel like I am walking a fine line in asking about what may be emotionally charged memories. However, sometimes when I ask the right questions, the most extraordinary stories come to light.

One such story came from an unassuming gentleman whom I treated in the late 1990s. His medical oncologist sent him to me when the only chemotherapy agents available had failed to shrink the more than twenty metastatic colorectal-cancer tumors in his liver. At the time we did not have many of the chemotherapy drugs or biologic agents that are now readily available to treat patients with stage IV colorectal cancer. Specifically, this man was referred to me to place a hepatic arterial infusion (HAI) pump that would deliver drugs directly to the malignant liver tumors through the hepatic artery. (For a brief synopsis on the rationale for HAI chemotherapy and on liver anatomy, please see the addendum at the end of this chapter, for those of you who are interested in such things!)

The referring oncologist informed me that his patient was a jovial, successful, highly respected, and beloved member of his community. I walked in to meet this man, along with his wife and daughter, who had accompanied him. He was of slight build, in his late seventies with brilliant blue eyes and a firm handshake. He maintained eye contact with me at all times in a manner that was initially unnerving. He spoke with an accent I couldn't quite identify, so I asked where he was from originally. He stated that he was Dutch and had grown up in Holland and had immigrated to the United States soon after the end of World War II.

I began to ask the usual array of questions about his cancer treatment and medical history. He reported he had been in excellent health throughout his life and had only been in the hospital once prior to his diagnosis of colon cancer. When I asked when that hospitalization occurred, he quietly said it was in 1944. I inquired why, but before he could answer his daughter blurted out, "Because he is a war hero!" My silver-haired, slender patient noticeably blushed and then shushed his daughter. Unfortunately for him, it was too late. I immediately asked him to tell me of his experiences in World War II and he recounted an amazing story.

During the war my patient and his family were members of the Dutch Resistance. His parents took considerable risks hiding people who were fleeing Nazi Germany. He said at various times they had anywhere from two to four members of Jewish families hidden in false rooms or passages of their home. However, he and his brother wanted to take a more active role in fighting the oppression they witnessed every day.

Late in 1944, my patient knew there were German munitions trains in the depot outside Rotterdam near his home. In an effort to disrupt the flow of these weapons back into Germany, he led a band of Dutch Resistance fighters to the rail yard. My patient, his brother, and four companions managed to dig under a fence and elude the guards. They proceeded to a train car and were surprised to find the door open. The rail car was filled with high explosives and artillery shells. They poured gasoline inside the train car, lit it on fire, and then, as he said, "We ran like the devil was chasing us!" After they'd sprinted a little more than a hundred meters, German guards discovered their presence and began firing at them. At that point, he stated, "All Hell broke loose!" The rail car exploded, knocking all of the Resistance fighters to the ground. There followed a series of tremendous blasts throughout the rail yard.

My patient and the other Resistance fighters looked for an escape route. Seeing an opportunity, they jumped onto a moving flatbed train car heading out of the rail yard. Unluckily, this exiting train passed directly in front of a guard post. German soldiers opened fire on the six men. Bullets hit my patient in the shoulder and the leg. His brother and one other fighter were killed.

The soldiers then pursued them on foot, and my patient saw another train rapidly approaching on the adjacent track. With no further thought, he ran along the flatbed rail car and jumped from one moving train to the other. Despite his wounds, he and the remaining men managed to escape. My patient was hospitalized briefly, but after recovering he and his comrades continued to fight alongside French Resistance forces and Allied troops.

I listened to his story, admittedly impressed by his matter-of-fact demeanor in recounting his harrowing experience. It was a remarkable tale of heroism. I asked if he'd ever been recognized for his role in this encounter. To my incredulity, his wife handed me a folder that included a picture of my patient as a young man in 1946 being awarded the Legion of Honor at the level of

Chevalier by Charles de Gaulle himself. The folder included a complete history written to accompany the medal describing the importance of the raid in destroying a large cache of weapons on train cars throughout the rail yard.

I read the account, mouth agape, amazed that this unassuming, quiet man had been involved in such an exploit. I would never have guessed that he and his family had risked their lives to assist people fleeing from Germany. I was impressed by his bravery in leading such a daring attack against a garrison of well-armed troops.

But that was not his last act of courage. Try to envision undergoing an operation that creates a six-to-eight-inch-long cut on your belly just below the ribs on the right side, removes your gallbladder, places a catheter into the artery going to your liver, and implants an approximately two-pound metal device slightly larger than a hockey puck under the skin on your right lower abdomen. After I explained this procedure and possible risks to my patient, without hesitation he said, "Let's get it done, Doctor. I have lots of living to do!" I performed the operation the following week, and he was discharged three days later.

After six months of HAI chemotherapy my patient's liver tumors had reduced in size by more than 80 percent. He continued to receive HAI chemotherapy, but two months later his liver became inflamed by the drugs and I told him we could not safely continue with treatments.

He accepted this information with his usual calm stoicism and reported that he would simply carry on and enjoy his life. He did exactly that for another thirty months and at every check-in he was always grateful and upbeat. He again impressed me near the end of his life when I saw him in the clinic, "I am a happy man doctor. I have lived a long and productive life and I have a wonderful family. Why would I ever complain?"

During his clinic visits my patient and I had many long conversations about his involvement in World War II. He was clearly affected by his memories and admitted that he was haunted by people he had not been able to save or help. I was awed by how he and his family had lived during the war, but more so by the man he was after his experiences. He was a man who had the courage and resolve to do the right thing and help others while combatting those who oppressed them. And he had the courage to fight a hard disease with dignity and grace.

I am truly fortunate to have a career that allows me to help people every day and to hear their stories. I am blessed to have cared for this man and many other veterans who chose to make a difference.

Addendum

In the decades leading up to the new millennium, we had very few drugs to treat patients with advanced colorectal cancer. Patients with stage IV disease, meaning the colon cancer had metastasized to organs like the liver or lung, were usually treated with 5-fluorouracil (5-FU) and leucovorin. These drugs generally did little to improve long-term survival for most patients, and dramatic responses rarely occurred.

One of the biological fascinations and peculiarities of colorectal cancer is that it will metastasize only to the liver in some patients. These patients may also have lymph node metastases removed at the time their primary colon or rectal cancer is resected, but in patients with liver-only disease, surgical removal of the tumors can be curative.

Unfortunately however, most patients have too many liver tumors, or tumors too near critical blood vessels or bile ducts, for it to be possible to consider surgical removal of the tumors. For that reason, I have been involved in studying other types of treatments to destroy or to treat the malignant liver tumors directly.

The liver is my favorite organ for many reasons, most of which are irrelevant to my current musings, but one interesting fact is that it has a dual blood supply. Specifically, the liver gets blood from an artery called the hepatic artery, which carries oxygen-rich blood from the heart. In addition, the majority of the nutrient blood flow to the liver comes from a large blood vessel called the portal vein. Everything we eat or ingest through our intestinal system passes into veins that flow into larger and larger veins, in a pattern like that of branches on a tree, until the vein-branches form into a single large "trunk," the portal vein. Thus, all digested food, medications, and other chemicals ultimately pass through the liver.

While the liver is unusual in the presence of this dual blood supply, it is like any other organ in the body when it comes to malignant tumors. A malignant tumor survives in the organ in which it originated or spread by a process known as angiogenesis. This means the tumor derives its blood supply from arteries feeding the organ. A colon-cancer liver metastasis obtains the majority of its blood flow from the hepatic artery, while a normal, nonmalignant liver gets most of its blood flow from the portal vein, with an admixture from the hepatic artery. Cancer clinicians take advantage of this feature of malignant liver tumors to deliver drugs or other treatments directly to the tumors in the liver through the hepatic artery. One such treatment that gained some popularity in the 1980s and 1990s was a device called a hepatic arterial infusion (HAI) pump.

Parenthetically, as a liver surgeon, when I consider removing malignant tumors from the liver I must always be mindful to leave the patient with enough residual liver to maintain function while the liver regenerates. The liver is the only organ in the human body that grows back after a major portion of it is removed. Clearly, the ancient Greeks knew this, as indicated by the story of Prometheus. His punishment by the gods on Olympus for giving fire to mankind was to have his liver eaten by an eagle every day, only to have it grow back, so he could suffer the same fate daily. Unfortunately, a human liver does not grow back in one day; it takes six to eight weeks!

3

Good News, Bad News

"The price of success is hard work, dedication to the job at hand, and the determination that whether we win or lose, we have applied the best of ourselves to the task at hand."

Vince Lombardi

Determination: The quality of being determined; firmness of purpose

One of the things I love most about being a surgical oncologist is seeing my patients for years after I have treated them. However, those visits are inevitably like the opening scenes from the old *Wide World of Sports* television program I watched on Saturdays when I was growing up. For those patients who receive good news during their clinic visit, the images are of athletes crossing the finish line in a first-place "thrill of victory." I tell the patients I am confident I can perform an operation to remove their cancer; or I confirm that their blood tests and scans show that tumors have not recurred after surgery, chemotherapy, or other treatments. Or

they pass some major chronological milestone without evidence
of cancer rearing its ugly head again. (Many patients still believe
the five-year cancer-free anniversary means they're "cured." If
only that were always true.) In contrast, "agony of defeat" scenes,
like the ski jumper falling off the end of the ramp and bouncing
hard on the slope, represent the distress and depression patients
and their family members feel when I deliver bad news.

I would never make it as a professional poker player because I
can't bluff when I'm holding a bad hand or keep from grinning
when I have a good one. My patients can tell by my face when I
enter the clinic room what the news is going to be. When all of
their blood tests and scans reveal no evidence of cancer recurrence, I walk in smiling and immediately tell them everything
looks great and I see no evidence of any cancer. The remainder
of the visit becomes a combination of medical checkup and social
enterprise. I inquire about the well-being of their children, grandchildren, parents, other friends, and relatives I have met. We discuss their pets, their gardening, their recent travels, and sundry
snippets of their lives. Patients frequently bring pictures of children and grandchildren, or travel photos of places they have been
since their last visit with me. Often they ask for medical advice
on conditions totally unrelated to their cancer as they get farther
and farther away from their original diagnosis. My patients also
know tidbits from my life. They ask about the status of soccer teams
I coached, how my son or daughter are doing (both graduated college and moved onto successful careers, thank you), and whether I
have progressed from owning a Ferrari lanyard to hold my medical
badge (I'm a fan of Ferrari F1 racing) to actually owning a Ferrari
automobile (I have not).

On the other hand, patients, family members, and my patient-
care team have told me that I am quite solemn when I walk in
a clinic room to deliver bad news. No "light-hearted" chatter or

discussion of recent family events or outings. The nervous, hopeful smiles on the faces of the patient and the family or friends in the room quickly fade as I describe what I am seeing on the blood tests and scans. Friedrich Nietzsche, the pejorative poster boy of pessimism, is credited with the aphorism, "Hope is the worst of evils, for it prolongs the torments of man." Thankfully, he was not involved in the care of people with cancer or other chronic illnesses. A particular woman comes to mind when I remember the importance of dealing with both the highs and the lows of delivering news to cancer patients.

The patient was the wife of an emeritus professor of engineering at a prestigious American university. Mrs. Professor had a grapefruit-sized, malignant, vascular tumor called an epithelioid hemangioendothelioma, or EHE, in the center of her liver. It's a mouthful of a name for a rare, malignant tumor of the liver. She had seen surgeons at several other hospitals in the United States and was told that the tumor was inoperable and untreatable and that if she was lucky she might live a year.

The professor contacted me, and I examined Mrs. Professor and evaluated her prior scans. Not only was her tumor in an unfortunate location but it was wrapped around two—and abutting a portion of the third—of the three veins that drain all of the blood out of the liver into a large blood vessel called the inferior vena cava. As a hepatobiliary surgical oncologist, I knew I must preserve at least one of these veins to allow blood that flows into the liver to flow back out properly. I ordered some additional high-resolution images to better understand the appearance of her tumor, and I realized it had a very thick fibrous capsule surrounding it.

I explained to Mrs. Professor and her husband that it might be possible to remove the tumor, but it would be challenging. Suddenly this lady who had been sullen, withdrawn, and tearful every time I had met her previously looked up and said, "If there's any chance, I'm willing to take it! I am determined to fight this cancer!" The next week I proceeded to surgically remove the entire left lobe and a portion of the right lobe of her liver. And I was able to gently dissect the tumor capsule from the third hepatic vein. The operation was successful and Mrs. Professor recovered well over the next several weeks.

The professor knew a thing or two about scientific investigation, statistics, and assessments of probability, and, having lots of time on his hands, sent an acerbic letter to the physicians at the other hospitals. In it, he explained in detail his mathematical analysis of the fallacy of their prognosis when considering an individual patient in terms of a statistical mean. He pointedly informed them that it was impossible to predict if any given individual would fall near the mean or several standard errors away from the mean. In plain language, predicting the length of survival of cancer patients is usually based on data from the life-span of a large number of people diagnosed with the same disease. Some people live for a shorter—possibly much shorter—time than the average, while others live significantly longer than the average survival time. The professor concluded, prognostication regarding cancer survival was imperfect at best—particularly since I had successfully removed the tumor (yes, he added that final detail in his letters). Unfortunately, for the next year, when I would encounter these various surgeons at national or international surgery or cancer meetings, I would get some frosty stares and very little conversation.

For the following three years, I saw Mrs. Professor every four months, and with each visit I would enter the room smiling and pleased to report that all looked good on her blood tests and scans. But three and a half years after her operation, the nature of the clinic visit, unfortunately, changed. The moment I entered the room the professor said, "Uh-oh!" Mrs. Professor immediately looked crestfallen and asked, "What is wrong?" I sat down and explained that there were new, small tumors in her liver and lungs. She asked how this could be possible since she felt so well, and I countered by informing her that small tumors frequently do not cause symptoms or problems that make a patient aware of their presence. I spent almost an hour answering an array of questions from Mr. and Mrs. Professor, many of which were different ways of asking me to predict the future and her probable longevity. I repeatedly explained that the tumors were a bad prognostic finding, and that her particular type of tumor was generally quite resistant to chemotherapy. She stated openly that she had no interest in taking chemotherapy or other treatments that would adversely impact the quality of her life.

She finally looked at me with tears in her eyes and asked, "Does this mean I won't see you again?" I immediately replied that I would continue to see her on a regular basis throughout her life and that, in my opinion, part of the job for all of us in oncology was to support and care for our patients through all phases of the disease, even when our treatments failed to eradicate the malignancy. I also confirmed that I respected her decision to decline chemotherapy treatment, and I would be available to assist her at any time. Mrs. Professor smiled wanly, and said she was relieved to know my colleagues and I would treat any symptoms and help her, should she develop any discomfort or other problems. I arranged for consultation visits with physicians from our palliative care service, and I continued to see my patient and the professor every three months for another year.

Approximately fourteen months after her cancer recurred, the professor called me and said that his wife was fading rapidly and they would not likely see me again. A month later I received a poignant and personal letter. In it, the professor included his wife's obituary from the local newspaper. It chronicled her impressive array of accomplishments and interests enjoyed over the course of a life lived fully. There was also a small hand-painted watercolor card from Mrs. Professor with a note to me. In it, she thanked me for giving her hope at that initial visit when I told her that it was possible to operate on her. She then wrote something I will never forget, "When I saw the other doctors, I felt rejected, trashed, and discarded. I felt they were dismissing me because they could not remove my cancer. All my hope was killed." The note went on to thank me for giving her several additional years of life to enjoy traveling with her husband, spending time with friends, and other activities that were important to her. I make no apology to Friedrich Nietzsche or his acolytes, for I know that the death of hope is a much greater torment for patients than the presence of hope.

Delivering and receiving bad news is difficult for everyone involved in cancer care (and any other area of medicine, for that matter): the patient, family members, friends, and physicians and members of the medical and nursing teams. There is an emotional toll on all of us. We can, however, deliver bad news with compassion and care, and that should be the goal. Patients have the right to know if they are facing a battle with cancer that they will ultimately lose, but they also need to hear a confirmation their physicians and other medical professionals will fight alongside them and support them and their family members.

One thing I learned early in my career is that patients may fear they will be abandoned when the medical community can no longer alter the progression of their cancer. Recall the words written by my patient, "I felt rejected, trashed, and discarded. I felt they were dismissing me because they could not remove my cancer." Regardless of the outcome, I believe we doctors must fight the battle side by side with our patients to the end, providing hope tempered with realistic expectations, compassion, and reassurance that we will be there to help throughout the process.

4

You Can't Make This Stuff Up

"Once we believe in ourselves, we can risk curiosity, wonder, spontaneous delight, or any experience that reveals the human spirit."

e. e. cummings

Wonder: A feeling of amazement and admiration, caused by something beautiful, remarkable, or unfamiliar

I was looking forward to seeing a septuagenarian patient of mine whom I expected to be my first true five-year survivor after resection of a Klatskin tumor. A Klatskin tumor is not some type of weird cancer, it actually defines a cancer in a specific location. Dr. Klatskin was the first physician to describe a cancer at the junction of the right and left bile ducts at the base of the liver where they join into a single trunk to drain bile into the intestine. (Bile is important as it helps the intestine absorb many types of the foods we eat, particularly proteins and fats.) The technical name for this type of cancer is cholangiocarcinoma. Most patients go to their doctor when their eyes and skin turn bright yellow from this small tumor that blocks the bile ducts, causing bile to back up into their liver like a clogged sink. If bile does not drain normally from the liver into the intestine, levels of serum bilirubin rise; it is the elevated bilirubin that imparts a yellow color to the skin and eyes.

The gentleman in question had presented with this yellow condition, called jaundice, and had undergone testing that revealed a small tumor blocking both bile ducts of his liver. The tumor was growing slightly up into the left bile duct so I performed an operation that removed the entire left lobe of the liver and a portion of the right lower liver. I also resected the external bile duct below the tumor and the back portion of the liver, which is called the caudate lobe, to assure that all cancer had been excised. The operation was complete when a loop of small intestine was brought up to the base of the liver and the remaining right bile duct was sewn directly to the intestine. This allowed normal drainage of bile into the intestine.

My patient lived on a ranch and had been a hardworking ranch foreman his entire life. He was lean and fit and came through the surgery and the postoperative recovery remarkably well. Few patients survive many years after this operation because this cancer has a tendency to come back in other areas of the body. However, this gentleman had been doing well on all of his checkups. I noticed he was on an upcoming clinic schedule so I was excited to congratulate him on five years of cancer-free survival.

Two weeks before his appointment his daughter called and said, "I'm sorry to tell you, but Daddy died." I was stunned; he had looked great when I had seen him six months earlier. He'd been vibrant and active, with no other·medical problems. I was concerned the cancer had recurred and we had not seen it on the previous scans. Still, I reasoned to myself, perhaps he'd had an unrelated problem, such as a heart attack or a stroke, that had felled him unexpectedly.

I stammered out my condolences to the patient's daughter, and then asked, "How did he die?" To my amazement, his daughter told me that two days earlier her father had been out working on the ranch as usual. He noticed a solitary bull in the field and for reasons clear only to him, he decided it would be a good idea to play matador. With several ranch hands watching, he climbed over a fence, took off his jacket, and used it as a cape enticing the bull to charge him. The bull obliged and promptly gored him in the leg, severing his femoral artery and vein. My patient had bled to death from a bull goring. How do you score that in your cancer-survival statistics?

I always provide my patients with a standard set of instructions when they leave the hospital after an abdominal (liver or pancreas) surgery. Walk two to three times daily; eat a healthy, high-protein diet (especially after liver resection when the liver is regenerating and using extra protein); drink plenty of water to prevent dehydration; and avoiding pushing, pulling, moving, or lifting anything heavier than twenty pounds. This last limitation is to allow the sutured closure of the abdominal wall muscles adequate time to heal and become strong enough to avoid an incisional hernia. (A hernia develops when there is an opening within an area of the muscle wall somewhere in the body and the intestine or some other structure pushes out. Many people know about a groin hernia, which is also called an inguinal hernia.) I ask my patients to adhere to these recommendations for at least six weeks after the operation.

One afternoon, I was in my office and my secretary informed me I had a call from a patient's wife. Four weeks earlier, the patient had undergone removal of the right lobe of his liver for a colon-cancer metastasis. I picked up the phone, greeted her, and asked if all was well. With a thick Texas drawl she reported that all was not well and that my "fool patient" had injured himself.

Before I could say a word, I heard her cover the phone and shout, "Come in here and tell Dr. Curley what you did!"

After a few moments' pause, my patient came on the line and said self-consciously, "Hi, Doc." In the background, I could hear his wife yelling at him to tell me what he had done to injure himself. "Well, Doc, you know how you told me not to do any heavy or strenuous lifting?"

"Yes, that's right," I replied.

"Well, I didn't," he said with a hint of defiance.

Once again, hollering from the background, "No, you didn't lift anything, but you just tell him what you did!"

After a longer pause, he astonished me by telling me I had failed to mention he could not use his riding lawn mower. Furthermore, since he had about three acres of yard and "grass don't cut itself," he decided getting on the lawn mower would not break my strenuous activity rule. As he was telling the story, it sounded more and more ominous.

"Okay, so you mowed your lawn on a riding lawn mower. What happened?" I inquired.

Thankfully, this conversation was taking place on the phone so my patient and his wife could not see the look of complete incredulity on my face when he told me, "I was feeling pretty good so all of a sudden, I decided to pop a wheelie on the lawn mower."

Now that was a phrase I had not heard before. I had popped wheelies on my bicycle as a boy, and I had seen trained riders do it on motorcycles, but never had I witnessed or heard of a riding– lawn mower wheelie. Flabbergasted by the unfolding saga, I waited. "So anyway, Doc, long story short, I fell off the back of the mower and when I landed I felt a ripping in my belly incision, and now there's a bulge there. I think I have a hernia," he finished matter-of-factly.

I managed to keep a calm and respectful tone in my voice and restrain my laughter. I asked the patient and his wife to come to my office that afternoon. Sure enough, Mr. Pop-a-Wheelie had disrupted the entire length of his muscle closure. Only a thin layer of skin stood between his bulging intestine and the outside world. I looked at him, shook my head, and stated, "Unbelievable. You just invented a new postoperative complication." His lawn mower adventure earned him a trip to the operating room that afternoon to reclose the abdominal wall muscles. I certainly never thought I would need to include "no popping wheelies on any vehicle, particularly a riding lawn mower," as a part of my standard postoperative directions.

Along with giving my typical recovery instructions, I ask my patients to avoid alcohol for six to eight weeks after a liver resection to allow regeneration of healthy liver. For one of my patients, this request was particularly problematic. He informed me during our preoperative visit that he was a professional beer judge. He had a regular office job during the week, but on weekends he would travel all over the country and judge brews in regional or national competitions. I explained that I felt strongly about the alcohol-avoidance issue, and he reluctantly agreed to abstain. As humans like to do, he reopened the negotiation five weeks after his operation. He called and informed me he had been given a singular honor. He had been asked to travel, all expenses paid, to Munich, Germany, to judge in an important international beer festival. Well, even I know enough about beer to know that a Bavarian beer festival is something akin to the World Cup of beer tasting, so I granted him permission to attend. However, I asked him to limit his overall consumption. He stated, "Don't worry, I promise I won't drink any more than one glass a day."

Three days later, I received an email with an attachment from the beer connoisseur. I opened it, and there was a photograph of my patient with his arm around a "glass" of beer that you could easily dunk your entire head and shoulders into. Technically, it was one glass of beer, and he had quite the grin on his face! It was a poignant reminder that we humans can be a devious lot and it is very important to be highly specific with instructions both before and after surgical operations. Now, I very carefully define reasonable activities and food and beverage portions for my patients to adhere to during their recovery period.

My operations are not limited to the liver. I'm trained to treat a variety of cancers in the gastrointestinal organs, anywhere from the stomach to the opposite end of the system, the rectum and anus. One unforgettable patient of mine was a prominent attorney, previously healthy and active, who developed a rectal cancer. The cancer was diagnosed after he kept noticing blood in his bowel movements. His primary internist performed an appropriate digital rectal examination and palpated a tumor. A subsequent colonoscopy confirmed the presence of a nonobstructing, biopsy-proven adenocarcinoma five centimeters above the anus. The patient consulted a surgeon who recommended complete removal of the lower colon, rectum, and anus via an operation called an abdominoperineal resection, or APR. Removal of the rectum necessitates a permanent colostomy on the abdominal wall, something no patient wants. My lawyer patient simply couldn't fathom the changes this would mean to his active lifestyle. He was in his early fifties and came to me for a second opinion.

We discussed a different approach; a course of intravenous, low-dose chemotherapy combined with radiation therapy every Monday through Friday for five consecutive weeks. After completing the chemoradiation treatment, his tumor was much smaller. With the tumor reduced, I then discussed surgical options with the patient and his wife. I believed there was an 80 percent chance I could perform an operation called a low anterior resection (LAR), in which I would remove most of the rectum, the sigmoid colon, and all of the lymph nodes in the area, but spare the sphincter muscles to allow control over the bowel movements. I would anastomose, or reattach, the left side of the colon to the small remnant of remaining rectum. Finally, because the irradiated rectum was at risk to leak and I wanted to give the anastomosis six to eight weeks to heal well, I would create a temporary ileostomy, a loop of small intestine that would protrude slightly outside the abdominal wall and drain into a bag. On the flip side of the option coin; if I found there was still tumor present in the short stump of rectum, I would remove the entire remaining rectum and my patient would be left with a permanent colostomy. I estimated there was a 20 percent chance this would be necessary.

He was not thrilled with these odds and presented a series of scenarios for me to consider in order to, and this is a direct quote, "save his ass." I returned each verbal volley and stayed on course; from a sound and proven oncologic-principle perspective I insisted on removing all cancer-bearing tissue, even if it meant an APR. After thirty minutes of presenting his case, my lawyer patient sighed, shook his head, and agreed to proceed with the operation needed to remove the rectal cancer completely. His wife was supportive, but after her husband signed the surgical consent forms, she made us both laugh when she stated, "Don't be a wimp, he'll do all he can to save that ass."

On the day of his operation, I was paged to call the direct number in the operating room where the procedure was scheduled. The circulating nurse answered the phone snickering and said, "You need to get in here and see something." Unusual, but okay, a little preoperative levity. When I walked into the operating room my patient looked at me, then at the nurse and said, "Go ahead." She pulled down the sheet covering him to expose his abdomen. There, written in large black block letters was the phrase SAVE THE ASSHOLE!

I was ready for him. I nodded knowingly, my surgical mask covering my smile, and responded, "You know, you are a lawyer. Most people think lawyers are assholes. Do you want me to save your actual asshole, or all of you?"

He roared with laughter, as did everyone in the operating room. Gesturing to the anesthesiologist, I said, "Put him out." As my patient drifted off into drug-induced somnolence, he chanted the same words written on his stomach. I got the message. Sheesh!

This tale has a happy ending, figuratively and literally. The LAR and temporary ileostomy procedure were completed successfully. As my still-snoring patient was wheeled to the recovery room, I walked out to speak with his wife. She smiled slyly and asked if her printing was clear enough for me to read. I thanked her for her fine penmanship and recounted the conversation I'd had with her husband in the operating room. She laughed joyfully, tears streaming down her cheeks, and hugged me and thanked me for saving both assholes. This couple was quite a pair of characters!

Six weeks after the lawyer's rectal cancer operation, I reversed his ileostomy and the flow through his gastrointestinal tract was returned to normal. I am pleased to report that the fine asshole, uh, I mean lawyer, is still alive, well, and cancer-free with all body parts functioning normally more than sixteen years after his sphincter-sparing operation.

Homo sapiens, we are an interesting species. Wonders never cease.

5

Opportunity Calling, Version 1.0

"The only thing that will redeem mankind is cooperation."
Bertrand Russell

Cooperation: The action or process of working together to the same end

Eight months after I completed my surgical oncology fellowship and was a shiny, new assistant professor of surgical oncology, it came time for the annual Society of Surgical Oncology meeting. Since I was the most junior member of the faculty and, thus, the lowest person on the totem pole, I was asked to stay behind to take care of the patients and "watch the fort." On the first day I received a phone call from my chairman. He explained he had forgotten that he had agreed to host a group of Italian surgeons who wanted to visit our institution before going to the meeting. I asked him when they would be arriving, and his terse reply was, "They are in my office now."

Okay then. I ambled over to his office and met a senior Italian surgical oncologist from Genoa and eight young surgical oncology

trainees from different institutions in Italy. We sat at the conference room table and spoke about management of various types
of cancers for more than an hour. I then led the entourage to
the operating suites, and we changed into scrubs. The nine surgeons jostled for position and watched while I performed two liver
resections. At the conclusion of the operations, we changed back
into our civilian clothing and returned to the conference room. I
answered questions for another hour, after which the senior Italian surgeon graciously thanked me for my time. All of the young
surgeons provided me with a copy of their business cards and I
offered a copy of mine in return. I thought to myself, "Well, that
was a pleasant experience," but I didn't imagine anything further
would come from it.

Three months later my secretary walked into my office and
informed me I had a call from Italy. I was mildly surprised as I
answered the phone and was greeted by one of the young surgeons I had met a few months earlier. He told me he was arrang-
ing a multidisciplinary gastrointestinal cancer meeting at his host
institute in southern Italy, and wondered if I would be available to
travel there to provide two lectures at the meeting. I calmly said,
"Let me check my schedule." I held the phone away from my face
as carefully as I could and tapped a few keys on my computer
keyboard for ten to twelve seconds. I returned the phone to my ear
and masking my excitement said, "Yes, yes I think I can make it."
I was sent requests for my lecture topics and my travel documents
and four months later I flew to Naples, Italy.

I was greeted at the airport by the young Italian surgeon who
had invited me to the meeting. I do not sleep well on planes so I
was a bit fatigued after an overnight transatlantic flight. This was
my first visit to Italy. I was a little drowsy until we began the drive
to my hotel. After the third red light we sped through, amid honk-
ing horns and flashing headlights I turned to my host and asked,

"Do most people not stop at red lights in Italy?" He replied, "In Napoli the stop light is only a suggestion." The harrowing car ride to the hotel erased my sleepiness, and my bags and I were deposited at the front desk. Mario Andretti, also known as Francesco, told me he would be by later to take me to dinner and would also drive me to the G. Pascale Istituto Nazionale di Tumori (the G. Pascale National Cancer Institute) the next morning. I wasn't thrilled by the prospect of further time in an automobile with this young maniac. Fortunately, the trip to dinner was very short, and I was introduced to delicious Neapolitan pizza. Conversely, the several mile ride to the hospital the next morning was more eye opening than the previous day's escapades, and I spent the majority of the trip encouraging my host to keep an eye on the road while I gripped the seat and door handle anxiously. I subsequently learned over ensuing years visiting other Italian cities and speaking with colleagues who lived elsewhere in Italy that even they find driving in Napoli a terrifying experience so I did not feel quite so cowardly.

Being invited to give two lectures at a national cancer center in Italy in my first year as a faculty member was an honor and a thrilling event. But I was also gifted with an important lesson from the adventure. I toured the hospital with my Italian hosts, and I noticed the large number of liver cancer patients there. Intrigued, I begin talking to the surgeons, medical oncologists, and epidemiologists at the meeting and discovered that hepatitis C infection is very common in southern Italy. I had been performing basic science and clinical research on liver cancer so I was startled to learn the number of patients they were treating on an annual basis. The epidemiologists there informed me that the entire Campania region of Italy is served by a single public health hospital, the Cotugno Hospital. Furthermore, by Italian national law, if you are a patient diagnosed with any type of potentially transmissible infectious disease, including hepatitis B or C, HIV, or tuberculosis, you are required to present yourself for a health evaluation at the regional public health hospital on an annual basis.

Eureka! Chronic hepatitis B or C infection is a common risk factor in patients who develop liver cancer. I asked the Italian physicians and staff if they were performing any type of screening or assessment to detect liver cancer in their large population of hepatitis-infected individuals. The answer was negative; they were not.

I delivered my two lectures at the meeting and then spent the next day and a half working with physicians at the public health hospital in Napoli. I recognized an unexpected opportunity to perform a clinical trial to screen high-risk patients to determine if we could diagnose this usually lethal liver cancer (the majority of patients who develop symptoms of pain, weight loss, or jaundice are diagnosed with advanced disease) at an earlier, potentially curable stage of disease in asymptomatic individuals. Together with the physicians and epidemiologists on staff, we wrote a protocol to screen individuals who were chronically infected with hepatitis B or C. The next year in 1992 we initiated our screening trial, which consisted of placing posters throughout the Cotugno Hospital. These signs informed patients with chronic hepatitis B or C that we would perform a blood test, a serum alpha fetoprotein (AFP) level, and a transabdominal ultrasound of their liver to assess for abnormalities suggestive of liver cancer. Our initial objective and hope was to screen a thousand patients over the ensuing three years. Notably and incredibly from my perspective, every chronic hepatitis patient underwent a core biopsy of their liver during their initial assessment at the Cotugno Hospital. This provided a treasure trove of pathology data on the presence and severity of virus-induced injury to the liver.

From 1992 until we closed the program in 2006 we overshot our goal considerably. We screened and followed more than 22,500 individuals with chronic hepatitis B or C.[1] Parenthetically, most patients diagnosed with liver cancer are not candidates for operations such as liver transplantation, surgical removal of the tumor, or thermal ablation of their tumors because almost invariably they present with cancer that is too far advanced to be considered for any of these potentially curative treatments. For this reason, in most countries fewer than 10 percent of patients diagnosed with liver cancer are considered for potentially curative therapy. Even among those who receive a transplant, surgical removal of their tumor, or thermal ablation of their tumor, only about half are still alive five years later. The average survival range is from six to eighteen months for all other patients who have more extensive cancer and are not candidates for a local therapy like surgery or thermal ablation. The primary objective of our screening protocol was to determine if we could diagnosis a higher proportion of high-risk chronic hepatitis-infected asymptomatic patients with liver cancer at an early stage, when surgical intervention was still possible.

We have learned, and will continue to learn, numerous useful pieces of information from our screening trial. First, we were able to diagnose almost 70 percent of patients with asymptomatic liver cancer while they still had stage I or II disease. Their tumors were small and not invading major blood vessels in the liver so potentially curative therapy could be offered. As a result, some of our liver-cancer patients have achieved long-term survival after receiving curative-intent treatments.

---

1. More than 90 percent had chronic hepatitis C.

Second, we learned that patients diagnosed with liver cancer came from a subset of approximately 20 percent of the total group of patients screened. The patients who developed liver cancer had a liver biopsy that revealed cirrhosis.[2] Therefore, the 80 percent of people who had no biopsy evidence of severe chronic inflammation or fibrosis (scarring or cirrhosis) of their liver caused by the hepatitis virus did not need to be screened as frequently as the others.[3] In patients with hepatitis C and cirrhosis about one-fifth were diagnosed at the time of their first screening evaluation with elevated serum AFP levels and/or an ultrasound examination revealing a liver tumor. Patients who had either of these findings went on to get a CT or magnetic resonance imaging (MRI) scan followed by a tumor biopsy to confirm the diagnosis and extent of the liver cancer. The remaining four-fifths of the patients who developed liver cancer were diagnosed sometime during their ongoing semiannual screening exams.

Third, we learned that new blood tests can be helpful in diagnosing liver cancer at an early stage. We discovered that serum levels of a novel biomarker, soluble interleukin-1 receptor, rose in liver cancer patients six to twelve months before AFP levels became elevated. We are continuing to study this and other novel biomarker blood tests in an attempt to increase our diagnostic accuracy. We recognize that we have a wealth of future data as we are following patients who originally had high circulating hepatitis C viral loads but were successfully treated with antiviral therapy. It will be critical to monitor these patients longitudinally to understand if there is reduction in their risk of developing liver

---

2. The overall incidence of liver cancer in the entire group of patients we screened was less than 10 percent, but the incidence in patients with hepatitis C and cirrhosis was almost 50 percent.

3. In patients who did not have cirrhosis, we reduced the screening interval to only once every three years.

cancer. Our cache of data will be mined for the next ten to twenty years to reveal additional findings.

One of the fascinating aspects of life as an academic physician is the opportunity to visit and interact with colleagues around the world. I have visited places I never imagined I'd see when I was a boy daydreaming my way through books about faraway and seemingly unreachable locales. I was blessed with an invaluable lesson from my first international experience. Now, every time I visit a new hospital in another country or around the United States where scientists and clinicians are interested in the multidisciplinary management of cancer patients, I inquire about the problems they face and the research they are performing. From our conversations we often identify common ground and potentially synergistic approaches to initiate collaborative basic and clinical research projects. Thanks to modern technology and communication in real time, we can perform large cooperative studies to improve our ability to prevent, diagnose, and more effectively treat cancer.

My first trip to Italy could have been nothing more than a pleasant diversion and an opportunity to enjoy Neapolitan pizza. However, as Louis Pasteur noted, "Fortune favors the prepared mind." The good fortune to perform collaborative and cooperative research that can affect and improve the lives of our patients is always an opportunity I want to seek. The data and results accrued in our Italian liver-cancer screening trial has led to several European Community grants to expand the studies to other areas of Europe. I have returned to the G. Pascale Istituto Nazionale di Tumori, which sounds even better when vocalized, many times in the past twenty-four years. Happily, more motorists actually now stop at red lights. And walking across the street is no longer like running an undulating, dangerous obstacle course. I will continue to visit occasionally to assess and review the amass-ing data. The opportunity opened to me all those years ago will continue to reveal new avenues for research projects in Europe and the United States.

And, the Neapolitan pizza is always worth the journey.

Molto bene!

6

Does Your Dogma Bite?

"Creativity is just connecting things. When you ask creative people how they did something, they feel a little guilty because they didn't really do it; they just saw something. It seemed obvious to them after a while. That's because they were able to connect experiences they've had and synthesize new things."

Steve Jobs

Creativity: The use of imagination or original ideas to create something; inventiveness

I like the silly humor in a scene from the movie *The Return of the Pink Panther*. Peter Sellers, playing the bumbling Inspector Clouseau, enters an inn to request a room for the night. After the usual language miscommunications between Clouseau and the innkeeper, the inspector stops and looks down at a small dog sitting near the door. He inquires if the innkeeper's dog bites, and the elderly man blandly replies no. Clouseau reaches down to pet the dog, which promptly nips his hand.

"I thought you said your dog does not bite!" complains Clouseau. "That is not my dog," calmly replies the innkeeper.

I love dogs. No matter how my day was at work, I have a happy homecoming when I'm greeted joyfully by my pack of pooches. Tails wagging, four dogs (Yes, four. I told you I am fond of them!) greet me as I enter the house from the garage, each jostling for position to be the first for an ear or belly rub. Frequently, a toy is dropped at my feet informing me it's time to go to the back yard for a game of fetch or rope tug. While dogs are great fun, playful, and wonderful companions, they can also chew your expensive new shoes to pieces or leave malodorous droppings in your house that you have to follow your nose to find. Dogma is much like this. Dogma develops in part because human nature likes to embrace things that are known, familiar, and comfortable. But dogma, like dogs, can be destructive or problematic. Dogma can suppress or discourage thoughtfulness and innovation. This is particularly dangerous in institutions where the leadership supports dogma and the climate does not advocate or encourage questioning of entrenched beliefs. In cancer care, dogma can be potentially deadly if we involved in patient care and research don't constantly remind ourselves to question the adequacy of currently available treatments.

In surgical oncology, dogma can develop as readily as in any other area of medicine. As a poignant example, in 1988 Kevin Hughes and others published a paper in *Surgery* describing the survival rate of patients with colorectal-cancer liver metastases that were surgically removed.[4] The authors reported that one-third of patients who underwent complete surgical removal of

4. Registry of Hepatic Metastases. "Resection of the liver for colorectal carcinoma metastases: A multi-institutional study of indications for resection," *Surgery* 103, no. 3 (March 1988): 278–88.

their liver tumors were still alive five years after the operation, most with no evidence of recurrence of their cancer. The paper is a seminal reason why surgical treatment of colorectal-cancer liver metastases, stage IV disease, is a common practice today, particularly since chemotherapy alone rarely cures these patients. For patients with colorectal cancer that has spread only to their liver, we can improve their probability of long-term survival by surgically removing or destroying their malignant liver tumors.

While this paper was very important in establishing the treatment of colorectal-cancer liver metastases, it was also responsible for creating surgical dogma. The authors reported that patients who had four or more liver metastases were less likely to derive a survival benefit from surgical treatment and, therefore, surgical treatment was relatively contraindicated. Because patients with four or more metastases had a *relatively* poor prognosis compared to those patients with three or fewer metastases, surgery was considered too high a risk for too small a gain.

Relatively is relatively open to interpretation, but when I was a surgical oncology fellow, this alpha dogma ruled. I saw several patients in the clinic who had four or more liver metastases that were technically resectable, meaning they all could be removed while leaving a volume of normal liver adequate for the patient to survive. However, we referred them to our medical oncology colleagues for chemotherapy treatment because they had "too many tumors," which was dogmatically believed to represent more aggressive, nonsurgically treatable cancer.

I think it is critical that we practitioners examine our patterns of behavior and our methods on a regular basis to stay on the cutting edge of treatment and to consider whether we can safely push the envelope to help our patients. As my fellowship in surgical oncology progressed, I went back and carefully reread the 1988 paper. In the discussion section, I was surprised to see that patients who had four or more liver metastases had a five-year survival rate of 17 percent, which was indeed inferior to the 33 percent reported for all patients in the series. This is what led the authors to recommend that patients with four or more lesions not be considered for surgical treatment. This confounded me because a 17 percent five-year survival rate was still better than the essentially 0 percent five-year survival rate in patients who did not undergo surgical treatment.

After completing my fellowship training, I decided that adhering to this dogma did not make sense to me. I knew my team and I could perform major liver operations with a low risk of life-threatening complications for our patients. I initiated a prospective hepatobiliary-tumor surgery database and carefully followed everyone we treated. For patients with stage IV colorectal cancer confined to the liver, I would consider surgical treatment that included removal of all tumors when possible. Or a combination of removal and killing additional small tumors with radiofrequency ablation (a technique that heats the tumors) when complete surgical removal was not feasible. These patients, like all our cancer patients, were then followed routinely over the course of their lives.

I tell medical students, residents, and fellows who work with me to question dogmatic practices and beliefs regularly. Challenging dogma certainly led to a difference in the lives of some of the patients I treated early in my career. In 2006 my partners and I published a paper reporting on 151 patients with more than four colorectal-cancer liver metastases that were treated surgically.[5] We found that 51 percent of our patients were still alive five years after

5. T. M. Pawlik, E. K. Abdalla, L. M. Ellis, J. N. Vauthey, and S. A. Curley, "Debunking dogma: Surgery for four or more colorectal liver metastases is justified," *Journal of Gastrointestinal Surgery* 10, no. 2 (February 2006): 240–48.

their surgical treatment, with just 22 percent staying disease-free. The remaining 29 percent who survived five years after surgical treatment had developed recurrence of their cancer but were still alive and receiving additional care. We learned the probability of long-term survival was improved using active chemotherapy agents before surgical treatment.

Importantly, my team and I are not alone. There are many surgeons and physicians worldwide who constantly investigate and look for better options to treat our patients. Around the time of our report in 2006, numerous surgical groups described their experience and confirmed almost simultaneously that surgical treatment of four or more colorectal-cancer liver metastases could improve the survival rate of patients. This goes to show that critical thinking and asking questions is in our professional DNA. We independently questioned Hughes's 1988 report, as all of us cancer clinicians want better results for our patients!

We can never predict exactly what will happen with any specific patient. Take two examples from my group of 151 patients. Both patients were treated in 1995 and both were successful professional men in their mid-fifties. One man had seven colorectal-cancer liver metastases, all in the right lobe of his liver. I cannot speculate why his tumors grew only in the right lobe, but that is what presented itself to me when I first viewed his CT scans. I removed the right lobe of his liver, which comprised about two-thirds of his total liver volume, and he recovered from the operation uneventfully. At the time of surgery he told me his goal was to see his three children graduate from high school and college. I diligently informed him that I could offer no guarantees and assured him I would follow him closely and intercede should his cancer recur. This year he became a twenty-two-year survivor with no recurrence of the disease. He attended his three children's high school and college graduations, and has gone on to see all three of his children married. He is now enjoying retirement, spending time with his wife, and spoiling his grandchildren.

The second gentleman's story does not have a similar happy ending. He had five colon-cancer liver metastases located in both lobes of his liver. I removed the tumors with a combination of wedge and segmental resections. During his operation, as I do in all liver surgeries, I performed an intraoperative ultrasound on his liver. This is the ultimate diagnostic tool for hepatobiliary surgical oncologists because it allows us to lay a probe directly on the liver and detect additional tumors that are too small to be seen on CT or MRI scans. In about 6 percent of our patients, we find one or two additional small tumors with the ultrasound that we did not previously see on preoperative imaging studies. But in this man, I found only the five tumors viewed on his preoperative CT scan. Like the previous patient, he was in the hospital for only six days and recovered uneventfully. Also like my first patient, pathology confirmed that all tumors had been completely removed with a good margin of normal tissue. This patient, however, represents one of the more frightening phenomena we sometimes encounter in surgical oncology. Unlike my twenty-two-year survivor who has never had recurrence of his cancer, I was shocked when I looked at my second patient's three-month postoperative images. He had six new liver metastases between one and one and a half centimeters in diameter. I was flummoxed because I had just evaluated his liver three months earlier with the best diagnostic tool available. While intraoperative ultrasound can detect small tumors, there is no device that reveals microscopic nests of cancer cells in the liver or in other organs. Clearly, the new tumors had been present in microscopic size when I performed his surgical procedure; I simply could not detect them. Unfortunately, his cancer grew at a meteoric pace, and he survived only another seven months while being treated with chemotherapy.

I say it to every patient: I cannot predict your future. Obviously, stories like my twenty-two-year survivor after surgical treatment of stage IV colorectal cancer are invigorating. The disappointment and angst represented by my second patient's story underscores the importance of continuing to push for more basic and clinical research, and better therapeutic combinations to improve the outcomes of our cancer patients.

Dogma can be comfortable and can lull us into a sense of security. We may invoke dogma to support decisions that keep us inside our comfort zone. However, I believe dogma should be questioned continually and comfort zones should be abandoned and demolished on a regular basis.

Probe. Inquire. Cogitate. Imagine. Dream. Attempt. Experiment. Push. Question. *Always question.*

"I thought you said your dogma does not bite?"

"That is not my dogma."

7

A Roll of the Genes

"Learning is not attained by chance; it must be sought for with ardor and diligence."

Abigail Adams

Diligence: Careful and persistent work or effort

Every week I have patients who will ask me about sequencing the genes of their malignant tumors. Or they will ask if their cancer is an inherited type because they are worried about their children and family members. Because there has been so much information published or discussed in the media, people are aware some cancers are hereditary. Other patients recognize that they may have specific genetic defects that can be targeted with a drug that normally wouldn't be used for treating their particular type of cancer. Scientists and geneticists have now reached a point where they can sequence the entire genome of a tumor, perform complete or targeted exome sequencing, or study a specific set of genes known to have a high probability of abnormality in given types of cancer. However, they generally find numerous mutations, deletions, or overexpression of an entire series of genes in most cancers, and these make it impossible (currently) to address all of the issues in any given patient's cancer.

Identification of specific genetic defects has produced major changes in the management of patients with cancer. A diagnosis of gastrointestinal stromal tumors proved uniformly fatal before it was discovered that there was a specific cancer-related mutation in the c-kit gene. A drug, specifically an antibody called imatinib, was developed that targeted the tyrosine kinase molecule encoded by the mutated gene. Now patients with this cancer can live for many years, frequently more than five years, even with metastatic disease. The same drug has been used to completely change the management—and improve the survival rate—of patients with Philadelphia chromosome–positive chronic myeloid leukemia. The publicized decisions of movie stars and other high-profile figures to undergo prophylactic bilateral mastectomy, because of mutations in their BRCA genes that portend an extremely high risk of breast and ovarian cancer, has produced more public awareness of the importance of cancer genetics. In gastrointestinal cancers, we carefully follow patients and their families who have specific mutations in the APC gene—which leads them to produce numerous polyps in the colon and, ultimately, to colorectal cancer. As with the BRCA mutation, when patients with these APC mutations are identified before they have developed cancer, we will recommend removal of the entire colon and rectum to prevent the occurrence of cancer.

I learned the importance of cancer genetics early in my career. A surgical colleague of mine from another city in Texas called to tell me he had a young patient in her late twenties who initially sought care for recurrent abdominal discomfort. On evaluation she was found to have a large pancreatic tumor that was determined to be neuroendocrine cancer. He was not sure the tumor could be surgically resected so he referred her to me. Almost as an afterthought, he mentioned that the patient was also having vision problems. She had seen an ophthalmologist, who noted that she had a partial retinal detachment and some small angiomas (small, nonmalignant tumors consisting of abnormal nests of blood vessels) in the retinas of her eyes. The ophthalmologist had suggested that this unusual situation is known to occur in a condition called Von Hippel–Lindau disease (VHL). It had been over a decade since I thought about Von Hippel–Lindau disease, so I studied the syndrome. Patients with this disorder develop angiomas of the retina, which can bleed and cause blindness. Among other things, they can also develop hemangioblastomas (blood vessel tumors) of the central nervous system that can bleed, leading to stroke, death, or, if the lesion is in the spinal cord, to paralysis. I found some notations that a few rare patients with VHL will develop neuroendocrine tumors of the pancreas or pheochromocytomas of the adrenal gland. Pheochromocytomas are tumors that cause abnormal amounts of norepinephrine to be released into the blood. Norepinephrine is the substance that causes rapid heart and breathing rates when you are startled or frightened, the "fight or flight" response. Abnormally high rates of norepinephrine in the blood result in dangerously high blood pressure, potentially causing headaches, stroke, or death.

I met this young woman and, after talking with her, I examined her, including her eyes. Even I could see the retinal angiomas. We obtained a CT scan that revealed a ten-centimeter tumor of the head of her pancreas that was encasing the portal vein and superior mesenteric artery, which meant it could not be surgically removed. We also identified numerous small metastases in her liver. Arising from islet cells within the pancreas, pancreatic neuroendocrine tumors can sometimes release high levels of peptide hormones such as insulin, glucagon, somatostatin, and others.

In this specific patient, however, there were normal levels of all pancreatic peptides in her blood tests, so she had what is called a nonfunctioning islet cell cancer.

I presented her findings at a multidisciplinary treatment planning conference. Because she had significant abdominal and back pain caused by the large tumor, we decided to try a nonstandard treatment. Radiation therapy is not commonly used in pancreatic neuroendocrine tumors, but we combined radiation with low-dose chemotherapy. At the end of a six-week course of treatment her pain had resolved. Because pancreatic neuroendocrine cancer is often slow-growing, I told her we would follow her closely and consider further chemotherapy only if her tumors began growing rapidly.

While my patient was receiving radiation therapy treatments I became a medical detective. During my undergraduate and medical school education I had seen family-history charts of individuals with a variety of genetic diseases. Depending on the type of inheritance pattern, the number of family members who are affected with a genetic disorder versus those who are not can vary. It's a bit like gambling; the probability of rolling a specific numeric total with two dice can be calculated, but on any one roll the dice may or may not show that total. VHL disease arises from a mutation in the VHL tumor-suppressor gene located on the short arm of chromosome 3 at 3p25.3 (the chromosomal address for the gene). The disease is inherited as an autosomal dominant disorder meaning that both males and females have an equal chance of being affected if they receive a mutated gene from either parent who carries the disorder. Recognizing this, I asked my patient's parents and her four siblings to come in for a complete evaluation that included MRI scans of their entire central nervous system and CT scans of their abdominal and pelvic regions. I was surprised by what I would soon learn.

The patient's father had no symptoms or findings consistent with VHL. Her mother had suffered vision problems for more than a decade, and our ophthalmologist found that she had numerous angiomas of her retina. Her MRI scans revealed she also had several small asymptomatic hemangioblastomas in her brain. She had struggled for several years with poorly controlled high blood pressure and her CT scan revealed tumors in both of her adrenal glands consistent with pheochromocytoma. Blood and urine tests confirmed she had extremely high levels of catecholamines, substances that cause high blood pressure when released in excessive amounts. Three of the original patient's four sisters were also affected by VHL, with all three having classic radiographic findings consistent with islet cell tumors of the pancreas. In two of the women, there was a solitary tumor with no evidence of spread to other areas; and only one had retinal angiomas. In the third, as in her sister undergoing radiation treatments, there was a large unresectable pancreatic head mass with numerous small liver metastases. None of the sisters had evidence of renal cell carcinoma (more common in VHL), although two did have simple kidney cysts. And only the mother of these girls had pheochromocytoma.

I dug deeper into the past and asked about any other family members who had vision or other medical problems. The mother of my patient informed me that her mother had lost her eyesight when she was thirty-one years old and had been completely blind until she died from a stroke at age fifty-two. This piqued my interest and I asked if there had been any tests done. Almost unbelievably, I was informed that an autopsy had been performed. I contacted the hospital in the small town where the maternal grandmother of my patient had lived and died, and after several weeks of phone calls and written requests, I received an autopsy report. Among other things, the autopsy described hemorrhage into a large hemangioblastoma in her brain that had caused this woman's fatal "stroke," and the report revealed that her blindness was caused by retinal hemorrhage and detachment. The mother of my first patient had only a single sibling and testing of this individual and her children showed no evidence of VHL disease.

After treating the malignant pancreatic neuroendocrine tumors in the original patient's sister, I performed a resection on the smaller pancreatic tumors in the remaining two sisters. Both recovered from their respective operations uneventfully, and during their operations we found no evidence of spread to lymph nodes or the liver. After treating the mother of these girls with the appropriate preoperative medical therapy for the pheochromocytomas, I proceeded to remove both of her adrenal glands, sparing the outer cortex of the left gland in an attempt to prevent her from requiring steroid-replacement therapy for the remainder of her life. Fortunately, the operation was successful, she never required steroid replacement, and her blood pressure problems resolved. Of the four affected sisters, only one had a child, and we found that he also had VHL disease. On his initial evaluation as a teenager, however, he had no evidence of any tumors either in the central nervous system or in any other organ.

We continued our investigative work with chromosomal-banding analysis, and we observed that the four sisters all had deletion of a significant portion of the short arm of both copies of chromosome 3. In contrast, their mother had a deletion of the short arm of one of her chromosome 3 copies but had point mutations in the other VHL gene. I love working in research institutions and medical schools because there are bright people eager to collaborate and provide insight and feedback. When I mentioned this unusual chromosome pattern to one of my colleagues, who is, interestingly enough, an expert in chromosome 3p (I guess the long arm of chromosome 3 was just too boring for her), she was intrigued because she had not seen this high incidence of neuroendocrine tumors in VHL patients previously. We obtained tissue samples from more than a dozen patients who had spontaneously developed nonfunctioning malignant pancreatic neuroendocrine tumors. Interestingly, we found that all had significant areas of deletion of portions of chromosome 3p. As we winnowed the findings, we discovered a novel neuroendocrine tumor-suppressor gene at 3p21.1 that was abnormal in patients with VHL-related pancreatic neuroendocrine tumors and in the majority of patients with spontaneous development of these unusual pancreatic malignancies. Because of the loss of a piece of the short arm of their third chromosome, these four sisters had VHL and were predisposed to develop pancreatic neuroendocrine tumors. This is an example of what we now understand after studying the entire human genome; loss or alteration (mutation) in specific gene addresses in our DNA can increase the risk of developing different cancers related to the genetic changes.

I previously mentioned that some neuroendocrine tumors can be slow-growing and that is true, but they still are malignant tumors. My first patient did well for just over five years but then began to show rapid growth of the metastases in her liver. We treated her with several different regimens of chemotherapy but she survived for only an additional eighteen months before succumbing to liver failure. The second sister who also had malignant pancreatic tumors fared better and survived for almost fourteen years before she, too, developed a large burden of cancer within her liver that no longer responded to chemotherapy, and she, too, succumbed. The two sisters whose smaller tumors were removed have not developed any new tumors in their remaining pancreas tissue and have shown no evidence of development of renal-cell carcinoma or pheochromocytoma. The sister with the retinal angiomas has had vision problems but is being treated aggressively by her ophthalmologist and has been able to maintain her vision for many years now. The mother of these girls eventually developed worsening heart disease, including congestive heart failure related to her years of poorly controlled hypertension, and succumbed to heart and kidney failure.

Cancer is genetic in that malignant cells develop because of mutations or other abnormalities that occur in genes. However, the majority of cancers arise as spontaneous, nonhereditary events. We know that environmental causes, including cigarette smoking or exposure to certain chemicals or radiation; some types of infections, including hepatitis B or C or human papilloma viruses; or poorly understood and undefinable simple bad luck can lead to the genetic aberrations that produce a cancer in a patient. We are in a remarkable period in cancer research because we may one day in the foreseeable future be able to target more of the abnormal genes present in any given individual's malignant cells. In the meantime, we closely watch our patients who are known to have a high familial risk to develop certain types of cancer, and we intervene early when possible to prevent the development of malignant disease.

It's an important lesson: preventing cancer is far preferable to treating cancer.

8

Told You So

"Service to others is the rent you pay for your room here on earth."

Muhammad Ali

Service: The action of helping or doing work for someone; an act of assistance

I love baseball. As a boy, in the 1960s, I played baseball every chance I got. My love of the game came from my father, who was a minor-league baseball player in west Texas when I was born. Like tens of thousands of other boys and men at the time, my baseball hero was New York Yankee centerfielder Mickey Mantle. In fact, the entire time I played high school ball I never went a game without my Mickey Mantle signature Louisville Slugger bat and Rawlings baseball glove.

Reading Jim Bouton's book *Ball Four* revealed to me the occasionally unsavory behaviors of my baseball hero. While my image of him was slightly tarnished, I still admired Mantle and considered him one of the greatest ballplayers of all time. In the mid

1990s word came out that Mickey Mantle was suffering from alcohol- and hepatitis–induced cirrhosis. He entered a treatment program and confessed he had spent too many years abusing alcohol and causing damage to his liver. He also admitted that he drank heavily because he assumed that, like his father and other male relatives in his family, he would never live past age forty. Mutt Mantle, Mickey's father, died from lymphoma shortly after Mantle's rookie season in 1951. Ironically, when Mickey Mantle was diagnosed with hepatocellular cancer his CT scans were sent to me to assess whether he would be a candidate for surgical treatment. Due to the severity of his cirrhosis and extent of the cancer, he was not. He went on to receive a liver transplant but died only two months later when the cancer returned in his lungs and other sites. I mourned the passing of an American icon and my personal baseball hero. I still have the New York Times front page and sports section from the day he died.

I have encountered many patients with a similar sense of fatalism. They have a family history with relatives who died at unusually early ages of heart disease, stroke, cancer, or some other cause. Their concerns about early mortality are understandable based on their own experience.

In the late 1990s a patient from a major Texas university was referred to me. He was a fifty-nine-year-old man who had undergone removal of a malignant tumor of his colon the year before. He then developed liver metastases in the right lobe of his liver. He was a bright, well-read, thoughtful, and charming man. He was a full professor and accomplished in his area of education. We discussed treatment options, including a right hepatectomy, the removal of the entire right lobe of the liver—which involves taking out approximately two-thirds of the organ. He had totally normal liver function and had been in excellent health otherwise so I felt he would tolerate this operation well. I also knew that the remaining left lobe of the liver would regenerate over a six-to-eight-week period, and his overall liver volume would return to near normal.

I always take time to explain to patients the features of liver regeneration, which is a remarkable occurrence in human biology. I told the professor that his right liver lobe would not grow back, but rather his left lobe would grow in volume and size to take over the function for the portion of liver that was removed. Many people assume that if I take out the right lobe, a new right lobe will simply grow back. They ask me if their right lobe is going to be a "brand-new liver." I invariably smile and clarify that the new liver cells will be mixed in with the old liver cells and that they will not reform as a normal-appearing liver.

I like to use an analogy based on my childhood experiences. As boys growing up in the southwest, my brother and I would frequently catch lizards, horned toads, scorpions, tarantulas, and other desert creatures. Every kid in the neighborhood knew that when stalking a blue-tailed lizard you had to catch it by the sides of its body. If you grabbed it by the tail, the tail would come off, and the lizard would scamper away and subsequently grow a new tail. The kid would be left with a still-wriggling tail in his or her hand—not as much fun as an entire lizard, but still good for disgusting your mother or the squeamish girl next door. I point out to patients that while I have met some folks with reptilian tendencies, the liver is not like the tail of a lizard and it doesn't grow back a new lobe. And I explain that after a major liver resection patients do experience significant fatigue for six to eight weeks while the liver is regenerating. That's because the liver is a selfish organ and uses a large amount of protein and energy to rebuild itself after a surgical procedure.

After a lengthy discussion, I asked my patient if he was feeling all right because he appeared sullen and contemplative. He told me that his father and uncle had died before the age of sixty-one. Therefore, he was not sure it was worth going through the surgery because he felt he was destined to have the same fate. He believed he was within two years of his expiration date. We had a lively conversation about the matter, and he decided to proceed with the operation.

I performed the hepatectomy, and he did quite well. Once he recovered from the operation and liver regrowth, he returned to his university duties. However, during subsequent follow-up visits during the first year, he had a somewhat pessimistic point of view because he wasn't sure the operation would make a difference.

As fate would have it, almost exactly one year after his surgery I saw him back in my clinic for a scheduled checkup and noted that one of his blood tests, a serum tumor marker called carcino-embryonic antigen, was elevated. His CT scan revealed a single new 1.2-centimeter tumor in the hypertrophied left liver. He was sixty years old. He looked at me and said, "I told you so." He had already received chemotherapy, so I encouraged him to consider a second surgery to perform a small wedge resection of this new tumor near the edge of the liver. I also advised him that this was a much smaller area of liver to remove and that his recovery period would be shorter. He went home to consider it and two weeks later he agreed to the procedure. Once again, he underwent the operation without any difficulty and his recovery period was uneventful.

One year later my patient went to the trouble of making an appointment on his sixty-first birthday. He informed me he did this to see if he had actually made it to sixty-one healthy. He was frankly giddy during the visit. He gushed repeatedly, "I can't believe I'm still here." We had a great visit and made plans to schedule routine checkups with blood tests and scans watching for any evidence of recurrent cancer.

I just saw the now-long-retired professor in my office last month. He is seventy-nine years old. He has moved with his wife to the site of his alma mater in the southeastern United States. He attends college classes in subjects that intrigue him and have nothing to do with his forty-five-year professional career. He enjoys playing golf and going to college baseball games. And several times a year he sends me handwritten letters and he includes newspaper and cartoon clippings he thinks I will find interesting. I immediately recognize his writing on the envelopes and I look forward to reading about his exploits and travels, and laughing at his well-selected cartoons and news stories. Every time I see him for a health checkup, we talk about baseball. I have shared with him my childhood fascination with Mickey Mantle and he admitted he was a fan of the Mick, too.

Each time my patient visits me in the clinic or sends a hand-scrawled letter, he thanks me for my care and for the additional years of life he didn't believe he would have. My reply is invariably the same: Always happy to help; always a privilege to serve.

I am reminded daily that none of us know how many days we will have on this earth. Things happen that are unexpected or unexplained. There are certain family tendencies or genetic disorders that can limit the life expectancy of specific individuals. Nonetheless, with our increased understanding of genetics and biology, along with the practice of a healthy lifestyle, we can change the fate we believe will befall us.

Unfortunately, cancer is a condition that will continue to trouble mankind. And sadly, too many cancers are induced by smoking, excessive alcohol intake, poor dietary choices, lack of exercise, and a long list of toxins and carcinogens in our environment. My colleagues and I are not able to cure every patient. Thus, an important goal is to find more successful and less toxic treatments so cancer can simply become a chronic condition patients can endure. As a society, we need to spend far more time and resources studying prevention of cancer, and that includes taking better care of our own health and the world around us.

We doctors always work hard for every patient, because we never know who will beat the odds and become a long-term-success story.

Like Mickey Mantle, I like to swing for the fence and try to go yard with each patient I treat.

I told you so.

9

The Five-Year
Cancer-Survival Mark

"Great works are performed not by strength but by perseverance."

Samuel Johnson

Perseverance: Persistence in doing something despite difficulty or delay in achieving success

Reaching the five-year survival mark after a cancer diagnosis is a milestone deeply ingrained in medical literature and in the minds of cancer patients. Problematically, many patients assume or believe that if they survive for five years after completing all treatments for their cancer, they are home free and "cured." The origin of the five-year metric dates back to the 1930s when surviving that long after developing most types of cancer was unusual. This predated the era of cytotoxic chemotherapy drugs, and radiation treatments were still neophytic. Back then, surgical removal of localized malignant cancer provided patients the best chance for long-term survival, but the lack of early-detection methods meant many people presented with advanced disease that could not be treated surgically.

It is unusual even now to read a clinical cancer paper that does not include five-year real or actuarial (predicted) survival rates. Every clinician involved in cancer care has seen thousands of graphs demonstrating the declining survival curve from the time of diagnosis until the five-year mark. Clinical trials for any given type of cancer are designed to compare a novel therapeutic approach to the standard therapy for that type and stage of cancer—with a goal of demonstrating that a significant percentage of patients live longer using the new treatment. There are many anticancer agents that have been approved for use because survival in the group of patients receiving the new agent was improved by a few percentage points (*statistically* significant when compared with the older therapy). For some aggressive types of cancer where five-year survival is still the exception, other so-called surrogate end points are now accepted in clinical trials. This includes measurement of "time to progression," meaning patients are assessed to see if a new treatment keeps their cancer at bay for a longer period of time, even if only a few weeks or months, compared to standard therapy.

I emphasize to all my patients that being alive five years after completing treatment for cancer is not a guarantee they're cured. Cancer does not read the textbooks and it can lurk in the shadows of various and—occasionally—unusual sites in the body. Still, cancer clinicians celebrate and love success stories. Eighteen years ago a woman in her mid-thirties presented to me with a nonobstructing rectal cancer and an eighteen-centimeter right lobe liver metastasis. The tumor in her rectum was bleeding and the large mass in her liver was abutting the right and middle hepatic veins, and was causing her considerable pain. When the medical and radiation oncologists and I finished her evaluation, we created a treatment plan that started with intravenous, multiple-drug chemotherapy for three months. At the end of that time, CT scans showed that the liver tumor and her rectal cancer were slightly smaller, and the patient reported her rectum was no longer bleeding. While unconventional at the time, I decided to proceed with an operation called an extended right hepatectomy, removal of the entire right lobe and a portion of the left lobe of the liver. The accepted sequence of surgical treatment at the time was to remove the primary (rectal) cancer first, then deal with the liver metastasis later. But, this lady still had a very large liver tumor involving two of the three hepatic veins, and if it grew just a few centimeters while she recovered from the rectal cancer operation, the tumor would become unresectable. So I attacked the liver metastasis first and removed the tumor completely, with negative margins. While recovering from this operation, she received a combination of low-dose chemotherapy and pelvic radiation therapy to treat the tumor in her rectum. This combination approach is used to treat many types of cancer, with the low-dose chemotherapy acting as a so-called radiation sensitizer, to enhance the killing of the cancer cells during the radiation treatments. After she completed five weeks of chemoradiation and recuperated for an additional four weeks, I operated to remove her rectal cancer and all of the surrounding lymph nodes. She recovered from this procedure and received an additional three months of systemic chemotherapy.

When I first met this young woman in my office, she tearfully showed me a picture of her two-year-old daughter. She stated unequivocally, "I want to see my daughter graduate from high school." I cringed internally but was circumspect in my response to her remark. I informed her that I would certainly do my best to treat her but I could provide no promises regarding how long she would live with stage IV rectal cancer. In May two years ago,

I received a high school graduation announcement from my patient as she celebrated the graduation of her daughter. I rejoiced that my patient had done so well and was alive without any evidence of recurrence of her cancer. For the next two days after I received that announcement I was energized and excited. Yes! A major victory!

Not every win can be considered an unqualified success, however. The treatments used for cancer can be dangerous and are associated with both short- and long-term side effects and toxicities. Consider one of my patients who has survived almost a decade after I removed the right lobe of his liver for colorectal-cancer liver metastases. His chemotherapy treatments included a drug called oxaliplatin because clinical trials showed that use of this agent combined with additional anticancer drugs improved the probability of survival. A common side effect of this drug is neuropathy. It can manifest as pain and tingling or numbness and loss of sensation in the hands and feet. This man is a cancer survivor who has never had evidence of recurrent or new metastatic disease. Yet he is extremely unhappy because he has suffered almost complete loss of feeling in his fingers and feet. Before treatment, he played a stringed instrument and was an accomplished member of a major American symphony orchestra. Now he is no longer able to perform because he does not have the sensation needed for the fine fingering work necessary to play in the orchestra.

Another, often-unspoken reality for patients who survive more than five years after cancer therapy is that the treatments themselves are carcinogenic. Many chemotherapy drugs and ionizing-radiation applications are mutagenic, meaning they cause defects in the DNA of normal cells. Cancer can arise in previously healthy cells decades after completing chemotherapy or radiation. For this reason, patients who have cancer as children or young adults must be followed their entire lives as they can develop second or even third malignancies.

When we doctors follow a patient, we watch specific organs or sites in the body, based on the specific type of cancer and where it originated, for any evidence of recurrence. Our knowledge regarding the particular metastatic patterns of different types of cancer was first described by Stephen Paget in the late 1800s. He recognized that cancers originating in different sites, such as the breast, lungs, colon, or prostate, tended to metastasize only to other specific organs or locations. This has been called the seed-and-soil hypothesis. Cancers that start in certain organs have a propensity to spread to other specific organs, much like seeds falling on suitable soil and growing successfully. For patients who have completed treatment for colorectal cancer, I tell them I will be closely watching the three Ls: the lymph nodes, liver, and lungs. Those are by far the three most common spots for colorectal cancer to metastasize, and microscopic nests of cancer cells that were resistant to chemotherapy can reside in those sites. Occasionally colorectal cancer spreads to the bone, but having it arise in other sites is rare.

Patients who have melanoma, lung cancer, or breast cancer will regularly have CT or MRI scans of their head because these cancers are known to metastasize to the brain. We do not normally perform such scans in patients with colorectal cancer because the brain is an unusual site for metastatic spread. However, as we have become more successful in our treatment of colorectal cancer at the primary site and in the three Ls, strange things have been happening. I have operated on more than 1,800 patients with colorectal cancer metastatic to the liver. Some of those patients are still alive and doing well with no evidence of recurrent malignant disease. Others have had metastasis recur in the liver or show up in the lungs or lymph nodes or occasionally as nodules in the peritoneal (belly) cavity. I also have an unusual, small group of nine patients who developed brain metastases seven to thirteen years after successful treatment of their colorectal cancer—after each of the patients had passed the mythical five-year cancer-free survival benchmark. Each of these patients was distraught and dismayed that the colorectal cancer had returned and all admitted they thought they'd been cured because their five-year anniversaries were behind them. The first few times this happened I was befuddled. I had not previously seen patients with colorectal cancer and brain metastases. In the past, patients with stage IV colorectal cancer had a low probability of five-year survival so the slow-growing cells that implanted in the brain didn't get a chance to cause problems. Nine patients out of more than 1,800 is not a lot of folks or a high proportion, but it is not zero, either. It is also not enough to change practice patterns, meaning I don't routinely order CT or MRI scans on the brain for my colorectal-cancer patients just because of these nine people. Sadly, none of the nine patients survived more than eighteen months after treatment of brain metastases.

This serves to emphasize the point I make to all patients; once you develop cancer you should be followed for the rest of your life to diagnose any evidence of cancer recurrence as soon as possible. Patients are the best judges of their own bodies and feelings, so I ask them to notify their primary-care physician or me for any new or subtle symptoms regardless of how long they have survived after their cancer diagnosis.

It may be time to set aside the five-year benchmark as a standard measurement of success in cancer care. With some cancers, including advanced pancreatic, lung, stomach, and esophagus cancer, it is rare for patients to survive more than a few years or even months. With many other cancers, however, it is now routine for patients to survive ten years or longer, occasionally requiring medical interventions such as surgery, chemotherapy, radiation treatments, or targeted therapies. Once diagnosed with cancer, patients and their physicians must remain ever vigilant because cancer could care less about statistics and probabilities. We must persevere and redouble research efforts to improve the survival time and quality of life of ever more of our cancer patients.

10

Opportunity Calling, Version 2.0

"It's not what you look at that matters, it's what you see."
Henry David Thoreau

Wisdom: The quality of having experience, knowledge, and good judgment; the quality of being wise

Liver surgery has something in common with real estate: location is important. Some patients have several tumors all located in one lobe of the liver that I can remove with a right or left hepatectomy. Other patients have multiple tumors in both lobes that require a customized, tailor-made surgery combining segmental and wedge resections to remove the cancer while leaving enough liver for the patient to survive. Conversely, and to the extreme frustration of hepatobiliary surgical oncologists, some patients may have a single tumor in a critical location that makes it unresectable. For example, a tumor nestled up under all three of the hepatic veins flowing into the inferior vena cava is usually unresectable. When removing areas of the liver, it is possible to take two of the three veins but one must be left intact to drain blood out of the liver. It is also crucial not to leave tumor behind on one of the veins (a positive-margin resection), because the cancer will recur and the patient usually does not benefit from a major surgical procedure that failed to render him or her cancer-free.

Patients with malignant liver tumors, whether primary (meaning they started in the liver) or metastases (meaning they spread from another organ to the liver), are frequently assessed in a multidisciplinary liver-tumor conference. This gives the team of oncologists, along with radiologists, gastroenterologists, and pathologists a chance to review all of the information on a given patient. Not infrequently, patients who have malignant tumors confined to the liver are not considered candidates for surgical treatment because the number of liver tumors is too great, the tumors are too large, or the tumors are spread throughout the liver in such a pattern that an insufficient amount of liver would remain following surgical resection. Or the patient's liver is cirrhotic, severely damaged, from causes that include chronic hepatitis B or C virus infection or alcohol abuse. Or the patient has the infuriating situation of a single tumor in a critical location where a negative-margin resection is not possible.

I was at a national surgical meeting in 1993 presenting the results from a phase I clinical trial using a novel approach to treat primary liver cancer. After my talk, two men wearing rumpled suits approached me. They explained they were engineers who had an idea for a new treatment for liver cancer. I believe I gave them a look akin to that of Mr. Spock from *Star Trek* with an arched eyebrow and an, "Oh, really?" They asked if they could buy me a cup of coffee. Since my serum caffeine levels were low at the moment, I agreed.

The engineers showed me a series of drawings of a type of needle electrode to be placed into a tumor that would kill it by heating it. They explained they had read my published studies about using new devices to treat malignant liver diseases and hoped I would work with them on their tool. I listened intently and then started firing questions at them. They were somewhat taken aback but quickly realized I was asking because I was interested. I inquired if they were ready to start human clinical trials using their ideas, but they explained they had only a prototype device.

This initiated a series of conversations between us over the ensuing months producing refinements in the radiofrequency generator and in the needle electrode. The design and composition of the needle changed multiple times as we explored metallurgy, tensile strength and insulation of metals, material malleability, and durability of the device. The final design was an eighteen-gauge insulated shaft with a series of sharp metal tines that could be made to protrude and retract from the end of the needle once it was placed into the liver tumor. When fully deployed it looked like the ribs of an umbrella. An electrical alternating current passed across the metal tines and resulted in ionic motion and frictional heating within the tumor environment. The goal was to produce heat sufficient to kill the tumor. This began my experience with radiofrequency ablation (RFA) of unresectable liver tumors.

After experimenting with different designs and materials, we finally had a prototype that I used to treat malignant liver tumors in animals. The RFA treatment yielded very high levels of heat, temperatures in excess of one hundred degrees Celsius, the boiling point of water. In our initial experience with the RFA device, the heating was so rapid the tissue around the metal tines coagulated and became an excellent insulator but prevented killing of the entire tumor. Thus, we learned to ramp up the energy slowly, over several minutes, to allow thorough and reproducible dissipation of lethal temperatures throughout the tumor surrounding the

RFA needle electrode. We also performed studies demonstrating that the treatment was safe and did not produce damage to other tissues or organs as long as they were not in contact with the area being heated. The procedure killed the tumor and a surrounding area of normal liver, which was planned and is similar to the way we include a margin of normal, nonmalignant tissue when we perform a surgical resection to assure no cancer cells are left behind.

Armed with preclinical and bench research data, I prepared a protocol to treat twenty patients who were undergoing surgery to remove malignant liver tumors. This is called a proof-of-principle study. In the protocol, I requested permission to treat one of the tumors intra-operatively with the RFA needle, and then proceed with removal of the area of liver that included any additional malignant tumors. Our pathologists confirmed that the tumor treated with RFA was completely killed as long as it was no bigger than 2.5 centimeters in diameter. Larger tumors required placement of the needle followed by RFA of overlapping areas of the tumor to destroy the malignant cells completely.

Confirmation of complete killing of resectable liver tumors in twenty patients led to a second protocol using RFA to destroy unresectable malignant liver tumors. The tumors were deemed unresectable either due to their location near critical blood vessels, which precluded obtaining a tumor-free surgical resection margin, or because of coexisting severe cirrhosis, which is associated with a high risk of postresection liver failure. Patients with primary or metastatic liver cancers were included in our study. The clinical research trials using RFA for unresectable liver tumors were performed in tandem at the G. Pascale Istituto Nazionale di Tumori in Naples, Italy, and in Houston.

In 1999, my colleagues and I reported our experience with

RFA of otherwise-inoperable liver cancers in our first group of patients.[6] We noted that the treatment was safe and produced no major side effects or toxicities in the patients. We also demonstrated that we completely killed the malignant tumors treated with RFA in more than 95 percent of the patients we selected. *Select* is a key word here as we were very careful to treat tumors that were not too large. We knew the zone of lethal temperature around the RFA needle was limited by the basic physics of heat dissipation in areas farther away from the electrode. This paper became one of the most frequently cited surgical publications in the world in 2000, 2001, and 2002.

During that time we continued to use RFA to treat tumors that could not be removed surgically. This included the use of RFA on small tumors in one lobe of the liver when we surgically removed larger tumors in the opposite lobe. We confirmed after treatment of hundreds of patients, even those with severe cirrhosis of the liver, that RFA could be performed safely with very low complication rates. A small percentage of patients did develop side effects such as infections, scarring around bile ducts, or injury to other organs if the practitioner using the RFA was not cautious in the placement of the needle. Based on our studies and those of other groups, RFA for unresectable liver tumors became an approved treatment by the U.S. Food and Drug Administration in 2001. RFA has become an important tool, used worldwide, to treat tumors that otherwise would continue to grow and lead to the death of the patient. I now have hundreds of patients who have undergone RFA of unresectable liver tumors who are still alive and doing well five, ten, or even fifteen years after their treatment.

---

6. S. A. Curley, F. Izzo, P. Delrio, L. M. Ellis, J. Granchi, P. Vallone, F. Fiore, S. Pignata, B. Daniele, and F. Cremona, "Radiofrequency ablation of unresectable primary and metastatic hepatic malignancies: Results in 123 patients," *Annals of Surgery* 230, no. 1 (July 1999): 1–8.

I recently saw one of these patients. When I met her in 2002, she was frightened by a diagnosis of an unresectable intrahepatic cholangiocarcinoma. She was told by her medical oncologist she would probably not survive more than one year. She was forty-three years old and otherwise in excellent health, and she had gone to see her primary-care physician when she developed some vague discomfort in her upper abdomen. Assuming she might have a problem with gallstones the doctor ordered an ultrasound of the liver. It revealed her gallbladder was completely normal but showed a tumor high in the liver. A subsequent CT scan confirmed a single eight-centimeter tumor in the center of her liver that surrounded all three of her hepatic veins. After additional testing, including a biopsy, it was concluded she had a malignant biliary tumor. She had been seen by several surgeons, and, like them, I felt that this tumor was not resectable. However, there was no evidence of spread to any other site in the body.

She and I discussed treatment with chemotherapy, radiation therapy, or RFA—which I explained was a newer treatment but one I believed was feasible in her case, using an open surgical approach. She agreed and the next week I performed the RFA operation. Treating a tumor that large required careful planning and monitoring with an intraoperative ultrasound probe placed directly onto the liver during the operation. I had to move the needle several times and produce overlapping zones of thermal destruction of the tumor. The RFA treatment took almost two hours to complete.

After the operation, the patient was up walking the same afternoon. She was relieved that I had been able to treat the tumor and was very hopeful that the RFA procedure had been a success. I was guarded when we discussed her prognosis. I explained that while I was confident the entire tumor had been treated, I could not be absolutely certain that there was not some small area of tumor still left alive. And it was possible a tumor that large could have metastasized somewhere else in her body. She listened and then cheerfully explained to me, "I just know that everything is going to be fine."

She was right. I saw her in my office a few weeks ago. It has been more than fifteen years since the RFA procedure. Her latest CT scan demonstrates a still-definable area where the tumor once was but where there is now scar tissue from the RFA destruction of her unresectable central liver tumor. She has never had recurrence or spread of her cancer. She is active, energetic, and, as she said, "living the hell out of life!" Hoorah!

A fortuitous meeting with two frumpy-looking engineers led to a remarkable opportunity. RFA has now been used on tens of thousands of patients worldwide to treat tumors in the liver and other organs. It is not a perfect treatment and it is not without risks or possible side effects to patients. Some tumors treated with RFA are not completely destroyed. Surgical resection and RFA of malignant liver tumors is a local treatment, which means it does not prevent cancer from recurring at another site where it is hiding. Regardless, RFA has allowed patients who otherwise would have succumbed to their malignant disease to live for longer periods, in some cases for many years.

Through all this, I learned a marvelous lesson: always listen to ideas; always look for new opportunities. The concepts may come from patients, family members, concerned citizens, inventors, research scientists, or medical colleagues. For me, when the concept came from a couple of engineers, something great happened!

11

Breathless

"A high station in life is earned by the gallantry with which appalling experiences are survived with grace."

Tennessee Williams

Grace: A divinely given talent or blessing; the condition or fact of being favored by someone

Cancer sucks. You may have seen the buttons, T-shirts, signs, or even Twitter and other internet memes bearing this proclamation. I first saw it when a new patient, a young woman who is the subject of this chapter, handed me a button and emphatically ordered, "Put this on your coat, and don't forget it!" Yes, Ma'am.

First, a warning: Do not read this story if you are looking for a happy ending. There isn't one. This is about the ugly truth of what cancer does to some patients and their families. There can be humor and amazing character that shines through an aggressive and painful cancer. But this is the dark side. I wrote the outline for this piece several years ago, but I have been hesitant to publish it. Some people may be offended or upset when they read this story. In that case, stop here. The patient who is the focus of this account asked me to tell her tale. She wanted people to know that cancer can strike at any time, at any age, and in any person despite the absence of genetic or other risk factors.

After receiving my CANCER SUCKS button, I sat down and listened to her for the next thirty minutes. It was not necessary to ask many questions because my thirty-year-old petite, fit, one hundred–pound patient provided detailed information about her cancer and other areas of her life that were relevant at the moment. To describe her as talkative is an understatement. She informed me she was a single mother, very busy working full-time and raising a four-year-old son, and she had recently earned a black belt in karate. She mentioned this last accomplishment several times during our first meeting, and then added that I should consider myself adequately forewarned of her martial arts prowess. Laughing, she said she expected me to take very good care of her lest I get my butt kicked by a girl. Duly noted, and thanks for the warning.

This energetic young woman had been enjoying her independent life, caring for her son, and indulging in vigorous hour-long karate sessions daily. For three months she had noticed an intermittent, dull right upper abdomen pain and backache. The discomfort was more pronounced after a karate workout and she self-diagnosed a pulled muscle. Two weeks before I met her, the pain had intensified and become constant. She visited her primary-care physician who examined her and realized her liver was markedly enlarged and tender. A CT scan revealed a large melon-sized tumor occupying the entire right lobe of her liver. A biopsy indicated the tumor was a malignant adenocarcinoma. Adenocarcinoma in the liver usually represents metastasis from another organ, such as the esophagus, stomach, pancreas, colon, breast, or lungs. The CT scan did not reveal evidence of a primary cancer at any of these or other sites, and mammograms, an upper endoscopy, and colonoscopy did not detect any abnormalities. She had no elevation in any of the serum (blood) tumor markers we measured, and the presumed diagnosis was a large intrahepatic cholangiocarcinoma.

When I perform a liver resection, I start with a so-called exploratory laparotomy. This is a full check under the hood into the abdominal cavity; the stomach, small intestine, colon, pancreas, pelvic organs, and kidneys are inspected and palpated. Despite her normal test results before the operation, during the laparotomy I felt a small area of thickening in the lower portion of her colon where it joined the rectum. I could not see any abnormality on the outside of the colon, but it clearly did not feel normal. I inserted a flexible scope into her rectum and it revealed a one-centimeter tumor at the junction of her rectum and sigmoid colon. It was a flat tumor and had not been identified during her previous colonoscopy. A biopsy confirmed adenocarcinoma. I realized I was not dealing with an intrahepatic cholangiocarcinoma, but a large solitary metastasis from a colorectal cancer. Leaving the colon tumor alone, I proceeded with removing the liver tumor knowing that if it grew only a little more it would extend from the right to the left lobe and become unresectable. During her recovery, I explained to my patient and her mother that we were dealing with stage IV colorectal cancer, and chemotherapy and another operation to remove the primary tumor in the colon would be necessary. My patient asked why I did not remove the colon cancer during the liver operation, and I explained the incision I had made was in the upper abdomen and her colon cancer was at the opposite end of the abdominal cavity, in the pelvis. I also informed her we had not completely cleansed her colon before the operation and it was possible she would have ended up with a temporary colostomy. I described what a colostomy would mean for her, and I admitted I really didn't want to get my butt kicked by a girl for giving her one. She found this answer completely satisfactory, complimented me for making a wise decision, and told me in resolute fashion, "We will beat this thing."

This remarkable young woman recovered uneventfully and subsequently received intravenous chemotherapy for six months. I then performed a second operation to remove the section of the colon bearing the malignant tumor and did an intraoperative ultrasound of her liver. To my disappointment, and again despite normal preoperative CT scans, I found two small tumors in the hypertrophied left lobe of her liver that a biopsy confirmed as metastatic adenocarcinoma. I destroyed both of these tumors with radiofrequency ablation, but I suspected that this finding did not portend well for her. My colleagues in pathology and genetics did studies of her normal colon, the primary colon cancer, and the liver metastasis but could not identify any known syndrome or genetic abnormalities that explained her developing colon cancer at a young age.

After her second operation, all was well. The patient returned to her home state and resumed her career, care for her son, and karate with joyous abandonment. She became my leading and favorite source for email jokes and humorous pictures. Rarely did a week go by without at least one hilarious, sometimes inappropriate joke, video clip, or picture from her. She also sent newspaper articles from her small town describing strange-but-true occurrences, and she would bemoan her fate as a diva living among rednecks.

I saw her every three months and all blood tests and CT scans were normal. But at the one-year mark the bubble of optimism burst. There were several new tumors in her liver. Scans did not show tumors at any other location so she received another three months of different chemotherapy drugs and then a third operation to perform a combination of resection and radiofrequency ablation of the remaining liver tumors.

One afternoon while she was in the hospital recovering from this third operation, I walked into her room with an entourage of surgical fellows, residents, and medical students. "I've been waiting for you and your team," she announced. "I want to show them what the mad scientist has created." Unashamedly, she pulled down the bed sheets and pulled her gown up to her chest to show an impressive combination of surgical scars and a new incision and said, "Ta-da, Frankenbelly!" She was a piece of work.

She agreed to an additional three months of chemotherapy reluctantly, noting that chemotherapy "cramps my style." Energetic and indefatigable, "Frankenbelly" recovered and returned to her small hometown. The weekly stream of jokes, pictures, and upbeat messages resumed. She also mailed crayon drawings produced by her kindergarten-aged son with the recurrent theme of a surgeon (me) performing operations on his mommy. There were unintelligible scrawl marks in the margins of the artwork, which my patient politely interpreted as her son's thank-you notes to me. She also told me he included warnings that he, too, was learning karate so I could be in for a double butt kicking.

Great. Double jeopardy.

Every time I saw this young woman she informed me she had a son to raise and her plan was to beat this "cancer thing." While I desperately wanted to be convinced that she could kick cancer's butt, her cancer never agreed. Six months after completing her third round of chemotherapy, her cancer roared back with multiple tumors in her lungs and in her peritoneal cavity and pelvis. Though the tumors in her pelvis caused severe pain, incredibly, she found ways to create humor from her own significant physical discomfort. During a clinic visit she described the pain as, "being pulled on my bare ass behind a BMW going seventy miles per hour down a rough asphalt road." She went on to explain she chose to be pulled by an imaginary BMW because she was a lady of class and distinction and she wanted me to remember that always. I will never forget her description and her toughness.

My colleagues in the pain-management service concocted combinations of medications to help relieve her discomfort. The powerful medications did not eliminate her pain entirely, but after about a month she reported that the BMW pulling her backside down the road had slowed down to twenty miles per hour. These words are severely overused these days, but this young woman was unbelievable and awesome! Her situation also made me feel an abiding sadness. The respect I had for her was complete, as was my admiration for her relentless determination and optimism.

Almost thirty months after I met this black-belt, butt-kicking diva, she developed a cough. A chest X-ray revealed that the tumors in her lungs were growing rapidly, and within days they almost doubled in size. She came in to the emergency room on a Sunday night because of coughing and shortness of breath. She was admitted by one of my colleagues in medical oncology, so I did not learn she was there until the next morning.

I went to her room, quietly knocked on the door, and entered. The room was darkened and the window shades were pulled down. Her admitting diagnosis was "difficulty breathing," but the reality I witnessed was far more graphic and horrifying. The awful image is indelibly etched in my memory and was incomprehensively brutal. My patient was wearing a large rebreathing oxygen mask and she was using every bit of her breath and energy to say goodbye to her six-year-old son on the phone. She knew she was dying. The only other person in the room was her mother.

They were both terrified. Her mother told me that her daughter had been struggling to breathe for the past six hours. She was taking forty to fifty short, quick breaths per minute. Despite the maximum oxygen flowing through the rebreathing mask, she was using all of the muscles in her neck, chest, and belly wall to gasp for air. She tensed and quivered as she made an exhausting effort to breathe. When she hung up the phone after a heart-wrenching conversation with her son, she managed to say she was scared.

I was surprised when she turned to the tear-streaked face of her mother and asked her to leave the room for a moment. Without hesitating, her mother left, and I sat down in the chair next to the bed and grasped her hand. She spoke, but it required more than five minutes for her to say what usually would have taken her fifteen to twenty seconds. She would gasp out a few words, then struggle for interminably long pauses to get enough oxygen, and then wheeze out a few more words. She told me she had said goodbye to her son and to her father. She had told her son that she would be there to watch over him during the course of his life. Then, after an almost minute-long pause, a noticeable sense of calm came over her and she looked into my eyes. "I'll watch over you, too." Stunned and stupefied, I stammered out an incredulous thank-you. She nodded toward the door indicating she was ready for her mother to return to the room. Her mother came in, sat on the side of the bed, and held tightly to her daughter's right hand while I sat holding her left hand.

My patient had signed a DNR, or Do Not Resuscitate, order the previous night. She did not want to be on a mechanical ventilator or have the medical team do anything to alter her invariable death. The oxygen mask was not sufficient to overcome the volume of cancer replacing her normal lung tissue. Nothing was going to change her outcome.

She glanced toward the window and I opened the blinds to the bright sunshine. As her mother and I watched, her fingernails, then her fingers, and finally her lips turned blue. Her rasping, maximum-effort breathing became slow, irregular, and ineffective. With a final pursed-lip exhalation, she passed from this life.

Benumbed by grief, after a few minutes I went automatically into doctor mode. I rose from the chair and felt for a pulse in her carotid artery. There was none. My eyes welled with tears that rolled down my cheeks. During the agonizing five-minute conversation I had had with her, she told me not to mourn her passing and to keep working to defeat cancer. But I did mourn. I also unprofessionally wiped the tears from my face with the sleeves of my white doctor's coat, and then turned, walked from the room, and informed the nurses of her time of death.

Grace. I have no other word to describe this woman and the gift I was given. I watched my patient die an ugly death, slowly suffocating. Her last spoken words were directed to me. I initially struggled to understand how I could accept such a gift in the face of her death because I had failed, and she had lost her battle with cancer. I eventually realized it was not my place to question such a gift, but to accept it with the dignity with which it was given.

The day after my patient's death, her mother telephoned my office and left a phone number for me to call, so I did. I realized it was my patient's cell phone when I heard her announce, with her usual buoyant, lilting, and teasing tone, that she was unavailable "just now" but to leave a message. I was initially unnerved hearing her voice until I remembered her saying that she would watch over me. I smiled and felt a sense of comfort, and I left a message. Her mother thanked me later for sitting with them in the hospital room during that frightening and difficult time. From my conversation with her mother I understood the source of my patient's spirit as she exhorted me to keep working to find better ways to treat and beat the disease that took her daughter's life.

As I mentioned before, this is not a pleasant or pretty story. But like the Taoist concept of yin and yang, it represents the balance of opposites in the universe. Light and dark. Love and hate. Conflict and peace. Beauty and ugliness. Life and death.

I am reminded every day of a basic reality: cancer sucks.

12

Mister Lobster Guy

"We ought to be vigilantes for kindness and consideration."
Letitia Baldrige

Consideration: *Thoughtfulness and sensitivity toward others*

"Hey, can you go find all of the medical students, residents, and fellows we have in the clinic?" I stuck my head out of an examination room and asked my nurse to go on a search-and-fetch mission to find trainees. "This is something they may never see again and I want everyone to take a look at this."

My nurse looked at me quizzically, "You want me to find all of the students and fellows and bring them now?"

"Yes, please go round up everybody you can and bring them in here!" We are in Texas after all, so rounding up people and cattle is something that occurs routinely.

Lest you think me a complete surgical lout, I will inform you I sought and received permission before sending out a

Calling-All-Trainees bulletin. As I was standing in the door talking to my nurse, the patient in the room was openly chuckling. He informed me he was becoming accustomed to these requests. He was a new patient, a previously healthy fifty-six-year-old man, referred to me to treat an unusual problem. He had carcinoid syndrome from liver metastases caused by a primary small-bowel carcinoid tumor. I put out the call to all of the trainees in the clinic because as we sat and talked, my patient developed a classic carcinoid flush. As I watched, a blush crept up his neck and onto his face and he turned bright red. I asked him if he was aware of the flush and he said, "Yes, I can always feel it coming on but I can never predict when it will happen."

He informed me he had been having five or six episodes daily for almost four months, and he reported abdominal bloating along with ten to twelve loose bowel movements every day. He noted, "I always know where the nearest bathroom is located." He had seen his physician after enduring these symptoms for three months. The inevitable, perfunctory CT scan revealed liver tumors and a biopsy showed metastatic neuroendocrine cancer cells. Further pathology and blood tests confirmed a carcinoid tumor, a type of neuroendocrine cancer. He saw a gastroenterologist followed by a medical oncologist and then ended up in my clinic.

This gentleman was a high school history teacher and his "events" occurred regularly during his classroom teaching sessions. He would turn bright red or quickly excuse himself for a bathroom excursion. He told me a great story. One day, he flushed in front of a class and a student blurted out, "Look, it's Lobster Guy!" The classroom went completely silent. In a moment of teenage angst that goes along with the sudden self-recognition that the brain-to-mouth filtering system has been disengaged, the offending student himself blushed red and mumbled an apology. My patient, a large, imposing man fixed the student with a stern look and stated, "Let me be very clear, it's *Mister* Lobster Guy to you." The class erupted with laughter and cheered!

A nickname was born.

After collecting half of a dozen trainees from the clinic, I had them examine his bright-red face and touch his skin, which was not warm. This is surprising because people who flush usually do so in the middle of a high fever and their skin is warm or even hot to touch. The students and trainees proclaimed "Oh, wow!" and "That's amazing!" and then quietly filed out of the room. I thanked my patient for allowing the teaching moment because carcinoid tumor and carcinoid syndrome are relatively rare occurrences in surgical and medical oncology.

Carcinoid tumors can originate almost anywhere in the gastrointestinal tract from the esophagus, stomach, small intestine, pancreas, appendix, or colon and rectum. They can also arise from the lungs as a condition called bronchial carcinoid. These sites contain enterochromaffin cells, and when they begin to grow abnormally they form a tumor. Carcinoid tumors have a predilection to metastasize to lymph nodes, and, for tumors in the gastrointestinal tract, to metastasize to the liver. Occasionally a one-centimeter or smaller carcinoid tumor will be discovered in an appendix that has been removed for appendicitis. In that situation, no further treatment is necessary. Or if a carcinoid tumor of one centimeter or less is removed during a colonoscopy, no further surgery is indicated, but close follow up and a colonoscopy every few years is recommended. However, for larger carcinoid tumors arising in the small intestine or colon, there is a risk of metastasis to lymph nodes in the area, so a more formal cancer operation that removes a segment of the intestine and all of the lymph nodes in the area is standard treatment.

Carcinoid tumors are unusual in that they tend to be very slow-growing, and many patients have them for years, if not decades, before symptoms or manifestations of the disease develop. For example, tumors in the bowel may cause obstruction or bleeding before a patient realizes something is wrong.

Carcinoid tumors are interesting because once they metastasize to the liver, carcinoid syndrome can occur. Serotonin plays numerous roles in regulating normal functions in the intestine and in the brain. But when excess amounts of serotonin are released by carcinoid tumors in the liver, the result is episodes of flushing, diarrhea, heart palpitations, asthma-like symptoms, and high blood pressure. If not addressed and treated, a patient can go on to develop thickening of the pulmonic and tricuspid heart valves and right heart failure.

I have performed liver operations on hundreds of patients with carcinoid tumor metastases and carcinoid syndrome, but I have never cured a single one. That may seem strange because a basic tenet of surgical oncology is to remove all cancer-bearing tissue with clear surgical margins during an operation performed with curative intent. Carcinoid is one of the rare exceptions to that hallowed convention. Patients treated with surgical liver resection or ablation techniques can live for many years, often for a decade or more despite the fact that the surgery performed is not "curative" (defined as removal of all detectable malignant tumors).

Patients with carcinoid syndrome from liver metastases have several treatment options available to them. Because their symptoms are related to release of excess levels of naturally occurring hormones that bind to specific receptors on the surface of normal cells, we can block the effect of the hormones with an intramuscular injection of long-acting octreotide in the gluteus maximus once every twenty-eight days. Octreotide acetate binds to somatostatin receptors on a variety of cell types throughout the body and can remarkably relieve diarrhea, flushing, and other symptoms related to high serotonin levels. My patients like to say, "It really helps the symptoms but it's a real pain in the butt!" However, this treatment is not effective in all patients. For many we are forced to increase the dose until we reach the maximum, and even still, some patients eventually develop severe symptoms despite the medication. There is now another monthly injection medication available that has helped, but some patients' symptoms are not totally alleviated.

We have had success doing nonsurgical treatments, including transarterial embolization or chemoembolization. For this procedure, a catheter is placed into the femoral artery in the groin and snaked all the way up to the hepatic-artery branches feeding the tumors. A material is injected through the catheter into the tumor blood vessels that blocks, or embolizes, these vessels and starves the tumor of oxygen and nutrients needed to survive. While this can be an effective treatment to kill large areas of liver metastases, the tumors are rarely completely killed by this approach. Chemoembolization includes chemotherapy drugs in the embolic mixture injected into the tumor. Clinical trials have shown embolization alone is as effective as chemoembolization for carcinoid metastases and had fewer side effects. This transarterial treatment can be repeated several times in most patients until they develop problems with the effects of repeated catheter placements in the groin. There are some new drugs that slow down the growth rate of carcinoid metastases, and even radioactive particles that attach to the cancer cells and zap them with a high dose of radiation. Like surgery, none of these treatments totally eliminates all the malignant cells, but they can relieve some symptoms.

Let's get back to Mr. Lobster Guy. I wasn't sure if his bloating and occasional abdominal distention were related to the carcinoid syndrome or to partial blockage of the small intestine by the primary tumor. I recommended surgery to remove the tumor in the small intestine along with all of the adjacent lymph nodes.

And because he had four lemon-sized tumors in the right lobe of his liver and one smaller tumor in the left lobe causing his carcinoid syndrome, I also recommended a right hepatectomy and radiofrequency ablation of the left lobe tumor. He agreed and I successfully completed an operation that removed approximately twenty centimeters of his distal small intestine with an anastomosis (hooking the two ends of the bowel back together) and performed the right hepatectomy and radiofrequency ablation of the solitary left lobe lesion. On the surface of his remaining left lobe I could clearly see dozens of additional carcinoid metastases smaller than a grain of rice. I knew I had not removed or destroyed all of the malignant cells but I had resected the vast majority of active cancer cells. After the operation, his flushing and diarrhea completely disappeared.

After a six-week recovery period and regeneration of his liver, he returned to teaching. I saw him three times a year with repeat blood tests including serum serotonin and chromogranin A levels (another blood test used as a marker for carcinoid and other neuroendocrine tumors). For more than two years he was asymptomatic and pleased with the results. He told me his students were mildly disappointed that he no longer entertained them with spontaneous and unpredictable flushes, but they were happy he was feeling better. Regardless, the nickname stuck.

I suppose I could have subtitled this story "The Many Returns of Mr. Lobster Guy." Two and a half years after his initial operation, he called to say that his flushing episodes had returned. He was now having two or three a day and had gone from having one or two bowel movements a day to five or six. A CT scan revealed that he had two three-centimeter tumors in his hypertrophied left liver. When we treated him with long-acting octreotide acetate injections and his symptoms did not resolve, we performed a hepatic-artery embolization treatment on him. This reduced his symptoms for only two months, after which he rapidly developed more frequent and severe diarrhea and episodes of flushing. A repeat CT scan showed that he still had only two tumors in the liver, but they were now almost four centimeters in size with some areas of necrosis (dead tissue) in the center of the tumors, probably related to the embolization treatment.

Mr. Lobster Guy made it clear he wanted to be done with the carcinoid-tumor symptoms and he requested a surgical approach. It had worked the first time. I operated on him the following week and removed one of the tumors near the surface of the liver and performed a radiofrequency ablation on the other. He had complete resolution of his symptoms within a week of the operation and was content with the choice.

Patients who have primary or metastatic liver tumors know after talking to me that a healthy liver will regenerate after a portion is removed. Often patients will ask whether it is possible to perform additional operations if new hepatic tumors appear in the regenerated liver. I inform them it is possible in select instances, and I have a few long-term survivors who have undergone two or even three liver operations for malignant disease. I also tell them the story of Mr. Lobster Guy. He is my personal record holder (not expected to appear in the *Guinness Book of World Records*) for the most operations on one person's liver. I have operated on his liver seven times. Just before one of my patients was to undergo his second liver operation I told him about Mr. Lobster Guy. My patient replied, "Nothing personal, but that's one record I don't want to break, Doc."

I provided care for Mr. Lobster Guy for almost fifteen years. Every eighteen months or so, he would develop between two and four enlarging tumors in his liver responsible for recurrent carcinoid syndrome. He steadfastly refused anything other than surgical options. On his sixth liver operation, it took me almost three hours to separate his liver from all the scar tissue in his peritoneal cavity. After a meticulous, tedious dissection to avoid injury to the liver and the organs and diaphragm stuck to it, I completed radiofrequency ablation of three liver tumors. As with all of his previous liver operations, Mr. Lobster Guy's carcinoid-syndrome symptoms disappeared. Inevitably, two years later he developed two new tumors high in his liver, just under the right diaphragm. I explained to him and his family I believed it would be very difficult to get to these tumors through another abdominal operation given the dense and daunting scar tissue I had encountered during the sixth procedure. I proposed a somewhat unusual transthoracic approach to reach these tumors. He was all-in and ready to proceed.

I positioned the patient with his left side down on the operating room table, made an incision between the ribs on his right side, and then spread the ribs to expose the right chest cavity. The anesthesiologists deflated the patient's right lung using a special dual-lumen endotracheal tube, a Y-shaped tube with one arm going into the right and the other into the left main-stem bronchus. This allowed the anesthesiologist to provide anesthesia and oxygen to my patient's left lung only. I performed an ultrasound through the right diaphragm and "Voilà!"—there were two tumors just under the liver surface. From there it was a straightforward, short operation to remove the tumors and leave a temporary drain tube in his chest to remove any air or fluid. He was hospitalized only three days after lucky operation number seven and was again free from his diarrhea and flushing episodes.

Mr. Lobster Guy was treated by an admittedly aggressive surgical approach over almost fourteen years. Other therapies didn't work well for him and he lived most of those fourteen years free from carcinoid-syndrome flushing, diarrhea, or other problems. In the fifteenth year of his disease, I admitted him to the hospital with pain in his pelvis and back and a partial obstruction in his small intestine. Scans revealed tumors disseminated throughout the pelvis and peritoneal cavity. His right kidney was not functioning well because a tumor had encircled and constricted the ureter, the tube that drains urine from the kidney to the bladder. I had a twenty-minute chat with my now seventy-year-old patient and his wife, and I explained this was not a situation I could fix with an operation. He nodded in understanding and said, "We've had a good run, but it's time to stop." I described other treatment options including chemotherapy. He listened politely, shook his head no and said, "I retired from teaching and I want to travel a bit with my wife and family."

For the next six months he did exactly that. I received letters and postcards from him from various destinations in the United States and around the world. The last note I received was from his wife informing me of his death from kidney failure when the cancer obstructed the ureters from both of his kidneys. She reported he had died peacefully without significant pain or discomfort, and most importantly with no recurrent episodes of flushing or diarrhea. He had given her a final message to pass on to me. He had always been a direct man of few words who had no problem making decisions to proceed with aggressive surgical treatments for his disease, so his final words were characteristically taciturn, "Thanks, Doc. Your friend, Mr. Lobster Guy."

I don't anticipate any patient of mine will break his record for most liver operations for malignant disease in a single individual. He was a unique, endearing, and unassuming guy. The unusual behavior of his tumors with only a few growing every couple of years is memorable. It was also interesting that medical treatments were not successful in him. One of the things I love most about surgical oncology, and cancer-patient care in general, is that we do not practice from a cookbook. Every individual is different, and the approach and sequence of therapies we use will vary from person to person.

Mr. Lobster Guy graciously participated in the education of medical students, residents, and fellows over the fourteen years I knew him. Whenever he came to the clinic with recurrence of his carcinoid symptoms, he would greet me with a bear hug. Being an educator himself and ever considerate of the usefulness of a teaching opportunity for my students and surgical trainees, he would say, "Go get 'em, Doc. Let's show these youngsters some blushing and flushing!"

13

What's the Alternative?

"As we express our gratitude, we must never forget that the highest appreciation is not to utter words, but to live by them."

John F. Kennedy

Gratitude: *The quality of being thankful; readiness to show appreciation for and to return kindness*

"Hey, Doc, take a look at this."

As I walked into the clinic examination room, the gentleman sitting in the chair stood up, gave me a warm handshake and then embraced me. He stepped back, and took off his baseball cap.

"Wow, your hair has grown back quickly! It's all the way down to your collar." I was impressed because only three months prior he had completed chemotherapy treatments that caused him to lose his hair.

He explained his rapid hair regrowth had occurred because he was taking a special cocktail of natural herbs daily, which he combined with a "smudge" of sage smoke.

"Smudging made your hair grow, huh?" I rolled my eyes, and we both laughed. Smudging is the burning of dried herbs and grasses to create smoke which is used to "cleanse or purify" people, ceremonial space, and ritual objects. This sacred practice is performed by many indigenous cultures to cleanse and protect the physical and spiritual body. I had never before heard it credited with hair growth, however.

I asked him when he thought it would be long enough to braid. This may seem like an unusual question for a male patient, but this man is a Native American who had had a hair braid down to his waist when I first met him three years earlier. He informed me another two months of eating and smudging herbs should be sufficient for his hair to grow long enough to return to his traditional tribal hairstyle. He made sure to tell me, as he does every time he visits me in clinic, he was grateful to be alive and feeling hopeful about his future. His simple thank-you is an example of a great gift I receive from my patients; it is always a blessing.

This patient first saw me with a diagnosis of a single colorectal-cancer liver metastasis in a difficult location. The tumor was almost three centimeters in diameter and was in the caudate lobe, also known as segment 1, of the liver. This is the portion of the liver immediately in front of, and draining through small vein branches directly into the inferior vena cava. Tumors in this location can be tricky to remove because of their proximity to the vena cava, hepatic veins, and portal vein, but in this gentleman it was possible to safely remove the caudate lobe and rid him of the cancer. He did very well for just over two years after the operation, when he developed three small lung tumors. He then received an intravenous chemotherapy regimen including a drug commonly associated with hair loss. Like many patients, as his hair started falling out, he chose to shave his head. Unlike most patients, he did so in a ceremonial fashion, in a sweat lodge with members of his tribe.

He had a remarkable response to the chemotherapy treatments and when I saw him back with his regrown hair, his blood tests and CT scans showed no evidence of residual or new lung, liver, or other malignant tumors.

After I shared the good test results and we discussed hairstyles, my patient engaged me in a dialogue on alternative therapies, a common topic among cancer patients. I learned early in my career that it is very important to ask patients first for a list of prescription medications they are taking, and then look them in the eye and ask, "Okay, now tell me what else you take."

My Native American patient told me that during his chemotherapy treatments he and members of his tribe would hold a sweat-lodge ceremony on a weekly basis. This included burning various types of sage and herbs while in the lodge. He also admitted to eating or drinking several herbal remedies and teas concocted by a tribal medicine man. I had asked him to provide me a list of the substances in these herbal preparations, and he complied with a page and half of various plants, roots, and tree barks that he added to his food or brewed as tea.

My patient was pleased but not surprised when I told him that there was a long history of identification and development of cancer medication from natural sources. Historically, Native Americans from the Pacific Northwest brewed a tea from the bark of the Pacific yew tree (*Taxus brevifolia*) and used it to treat a number of maladies, including skin and other types of cancer, arthritis, and even the common cold. In the 1960s, teams from the U.S. Department of Agriculture collected botanical specimens from many species of plants and trees and provided them to the National Cancer Institute. The National Cancer Institute was performing studies looking for any naturally occurring compounds with anticancer activity. The Pacific yew tree proved to be a source of the now widely used drug Paclitaxel. Thus, there was a chemical and pharmaceutical validation that teas made from the bark of the Pacific yew tree actually could have anticancer activity. I mentioned to my patient that finding Paclitaxel in the bark of the slow-growing yew tree had, however, produced a firestorm because conservationists feared overharvesting the tree would lead to its extinction. The original production process required more than twenty-four pounds of bark to manufacture only half a gram of the active chemotherapy drug. Harvesting the yew trees for this purpose would have led to the destruction of old-growth Pacific Northwest forests. Fortunately, the pharmaceutical industry discovered alternative techniques to produce the drug and spared the dwindling population of trees. My patient nodded as I recounted this story. He noted Native Americans respect the land and the world around them, and the destruction of many of our forests, grasslands, and natural resources is a source of great sadness for him.

Native Americans are not the only group that commonly uses natural remedies. No doubt social anthropologists have found many cultures, historic or current, whose members apply natural substances as poultices or ingest medications to treat illness. The woman who lived next door to one of my aunts when I was a child was a Hispanic *curandera*. *Curanderas* and *curanderos* are healers who recommend, and often mix, a variety of natural animal- and plant-based remedies for just about any type of malady you can imagine. This includes preparations for headaches, sinus problems, influenza, cancer, and even depression when your girlfriend or boyfriend breaks up with you. I learned about this last potion when my then–high school–aged cousin was upset over a romance gone sour. However, he decided not to drink the brew prescribed by his neighborhood *curandera* and simply got on with his life.

Probably a good decision.

I get a variety of responses from patients when I ask them what nonprescription drugs or natural remedies they are taking. Some provide a list readily, while others are evasive, uncertain as to why I am asking the question. I always inform them it is important that I know all agents they take during their cancer care. Interestingly, some compounds may have some beneficial effects, including stimulation of immune function during standard chemotherapy. (Anticancer drugs can moderately to severely impair immune-system functions, increasing the risk of serious, even life-threatening, infections.) On the flip side of the coin, some herbal preparations and natural remedies can have an adverse impact and may cause dangerously high blood pressure during chemotherapy treatments or during the anesthesia used for cancer operations. Others act as anticoagulants and cause excessive bleeding, which is highly problematic and undesirable during a surgical procedure. I am not opposed to patients' using alternative therapies, but I do want to be certain we are safe in our approach to their treatment. I do warn patients to be wary of spectacular claims of unsubstantiated cancer cures from rogues, charlatans, and predatory miscreants. People facing a frightening and potentially lethal cancer diagnosis can fall prey to unscrupulous quacks. When patients ask my opinion about using alternative therapies, whether it is a specific substance or just their use in general, I utter a common truism: if it sounds too good to be true, it probably is.

In the cancer-treatment community, we really don't know how many patients add so-called complementary and alternative therapies into their prescribed treatment programs. Though the question has been asked and studied, the results vary depending on the definition of *alternative medications* and the veracity of patients who may not be willing to admit they are taking nontraditional substances or treatments. I frequently receive email queries or am asked by patients, family members, and friends about agents or equipment someone recommended or they found during an internet search regarding better or less toxic treatments for cancer. I do not discourage this practice and I actually provide patients with a list of resources including reputable academic institutions and individuals who are performing active research on alternative therapies and drugs. Thankfully, the National Cancer Institute and other research bodies have recognized that naturally occurring substances can have biologic and medical activity.

The fact is, a significant portion of cancer patients take nonprescription medications while receiving traditional cancer therapies. Frankly, most of these nonprescription therapies are innocuous and produce neither harm nor benefit. Some may actually have a positive effect and improve immune function, appetite, nutritional status, or the difficult-to-measure mental well-being of the patient. But, sadly, there are documented examples of patients' suffering serious side effects or even dying from using alternative approaches. Some patients who favor alternative treatments in lieu of standard therapies may have a shorter survival time when their cancer progresses rapidly.

A series of factors, including fear, hope, uncertainty, and a desire to try everything possible to improve the odds of defeating cancer leads patients to try all kinds of nonprescribed therapies. In my opinion, however, it is a mistake for medical professionals to denigrate or disdain alternative therapies because that attitude fails to recognize that most patients want to have input in their cancer treatments. I prefer to engage my patients in an open and honest conversation about all therapies they are using as part of their cancer treatment. It provides them reassurance that we can have an open-minded dialogue about all components of their cancer care. Sometimes I learn new and important information myself. Generally, I am able to validate that the tablets, teas, concoctions, or contraptions they are using are not toxic and may provide some unmeasurable benefit, and other times I can warn them when I find they are taking a substance or using a device that is dangerous.

It is impossible to measure the potency of hope and comfort that patients and families derive from trying everything they believe may help improve their chances of surviving a battle with cancer. Hope endures. And you can't write a prescription for hope.

14

Go for It

"By having a reverence for life, we enter into a spiritual relation with the world. By practicing reverence for life we become good, deep, and alive."

Albert Schweitzer

Reverence: Deep respect for someone or something

How long does it take you to make a decision about a major purchase? For example, a new car. Most people I know or have observed use a significant amount of time evaluating different manufacturers and models. Their research and calculated considerations include questions like, Do I go with a gas-guzzling SUV or an extended–crew cab truck certain to protrude a few feet into the parking lot driving lanes? Or am I feeling eco-friendly? Do I go with a hybrid vehicle? I was once a member of the Sierra Club, perhaps I should go totally electric. How far can I drive on a single full charge of the batteries in one of those things? And where do I plug it in once I reach my destination? People consider option packages and colors of the exterior and interior.

They take different cars for test drives and consult the internet or consumer-information sources to learn which are the safest and most reliable. I daresay we humans will take hours, days, or weeks to come to a final conclusion before signing a contract for a new automobile.

A stark contrast is our response to well-placed, impulse-buy items at the ends of the aisles in department stores or near the checkout counter at the local supermarket. Trinkets, baubles, gadgets, flashlights, batteries, gum, candy, and magazines with titillating sagas about the woes befalling various celebrities are placed strategically to catch the shoppers' (or their children's) eye. Clearly, businesses have done market research on the spontaneous buying habits of the average consumer. We apparently don't mind spending a couple of bucks on an item we may or may not actually need. Do I have enough AA batteries? Can I own too many flashlights? It has been a few days since I treated myself to my favorite candy bar so certainly another is a good idea. Poor impulse control + ready access to excess fat and carbohydrates = an increasingly obese population.

What astonishes me, however, is how little time it takes to discuss and convince a patient that a major surgical operation is indicated. This should not represent an impulsive decision-making situation. I realize there are caveats and disclaimers to be considered. The great majority of patients I evaluate for a surgical procedure are dealing with a diagnosis of cancer. Patients are educated and well informed enough to understand that for most solid tumors, surgery is a critical and established component of cancer treatment. Patients know from personal experience with friends or family that surgical removal of cancer is known to yield a chance for cure in subsets of patients, particularly those with early-stage disease confined to the organ of origin, that is, disease that has not spread to regional lymph nodes or other organs. People are still frightened about cytotoxic chemotherapy or ionizing-radiation treatments, and their fear is usually based on witnessed or recounted horror stories about terrible side effects and the painful demise of someone they knew. Yet when I walk into an examination room to discuss the details of a proposed surgical procedure I am frequently told, "I trust you, Doc, just cut it out. Tomorrow, if possible." I cannot begin to count the number of times I have heard the three words that sound like a slogan for an athletic shoe and apparel company, "Go for it!"

Evaluating a new patient for surgical treatment of a malignant disease starts with the patient's history and physical examination. The surgeon, or an individual designated by the surgeon such as a physician's assistant, nurse practitioner, surgical resident, or surgical oncology fellow will query the patient about how he or she came to be diagnosed with a malignant disease. The practitioner obtains patient information about any other medical issues such as high blood pressure, heart problems, or diabetes, along with a history of all prior surgical procedures and response to anesthesia and pain medications. A thorough review of all body systems is noted (akin to a preflight checklist to assure that everything is green and good to go before take-off on an airplane flight), and a complete list of allergies and current medications is recorded. Personal habits such as cigarette smoking, alcohol consumption, and any previous illicit drug use are solicited. After completing the medical history, the patient's vital signs (blood pressure, pulse rate, breathing rate, weight and height) are measured, and then a physical examination including visual inspection and manual palpation of the head and neck region, back, chest, and arms and legs is performed. The examiner listens to the patient's lungs and heart with a stethoscope, pokes and prods the patient's abdomen, and explores the lymph node–bearing regions in the neck, under the arms, and in the groin by touch. And if the physician is really thorough, a rectal examination is performed. This is particularly relevant if the patient is being evaluated for a gastrointestinal, genitourinary, or gynecological malignancy because the surgeon wants to determine if there is any trace of blood present and if a tumor can be palpated with the probing finger.

After completing the history and physical examination, the surgeon reviews the results of any biopsies already performed on the tumor(s) and looks at CT or MRI results. If the patient has not yet had a biopsy or undergone adequate radiographic evaluation, the surgeon orders such tests and reviews the subsequent results with the patient and the patient's family members at a follow-up visit. Finally, it is time to discuss an operation.

This is when things become surprising to me. I am primarily a hepatobiliary surgical oncologist. The majority of patients I operate on have stage IV cancer that has spread from organs like the colon, rectum, breasts, or other sites to the liver. Some patients have a primary cancer like hepatocellular carcinoma or cholangiocarcinoma that has arisen in the liver. To employ the vernacular, a liver resection is a big deal. Frankly, most cancer operations are major surgical procedures, and even relatively minor surgical oncology operations are not without risks or possible complications. Yet, despite the complexities associated with a liver resection and the mandatory discussion of potential risks, complications, and alternatives, the average conversation to reach an agreement to schedule an operation takes less than ten minutes. An average is an average, meaning some conversations are shorter and some are longer. Some patients literally tell me, "I don't want to know anything about the operation, I just want the cancer out." I insist on describing the steps of the operation and the potential complications, but at times patients respond by shaking their head with an emphatic "No!" They ask for the consent form to sign and tell me to proceed at flank speed.

Sorry, not going to happen, they must at least listen to my basic recitation about the operation. For all my patients I use pictures and artwork of the liver to describe the location of their liver tumor or tumors, and to define the areas to be surgically removed. Even for those not wanting to hear it, I mention a frightening list of potential complications associated with major liver operations. Most patients listen intently and nod, and may ask only one or two questions.

At times I do come across patients who are prepared with pages of written questions on which they dutifully jot down my responses. They request detailed descriptions of surgical techniques and diagrams of liver anatomy. We discuss the regenerative capacity of the liver and the probability of various complications during or after the operation. Often they will leave to consult with family, friends, the internet, and other physicians. We agree to meet again or arrange a phone conversation to discuss their decision. However, this ask-lots-of-questions-and-take-a-long-time-to-decide group is a small minority of the patients I meet. Usually when I ask the patients and those accompanying them if they have any questions, the answer is no or a simple remark such as "I trust you and I just want to get this taken care of." The other frequent comment I hear is, "I am putting my life in your hands."

In my hands. No pressure, right? That is a heavy load of responsibility and belief in my abilities laid at my feet. It is a burden all surgeons and physicians pick up and carry every day of their professional lives.

Trust is not something to take lightly or dismiss. It is an honor and a tremendous responsibility for surgeons to be granted such faith in their abilities and care. We are accorded a remarkable degree of respect and deference for our training, commitment, and willingness to attack and seek to eradicate our patients' malignant disease. At the same time, we want to achieve this goal without causing long-term side effects or problems for our patients. The trust is sacred to me; I feel an abiding obligation to all of my patients who believe in my skill and entrust me with their lives.

It is common for patients to ask for a prediction of the future. Many patients or a family member (the latter occasionally to the considerable annoyance of the patient) will have done research on their own. They have read about short- and long-term probabilities of survival with their particular type of cancer. How long any specific patient will survive is an impossible question to answer, but it's one I get every week in the clinic. My overused line is to tell people that I do not have a crystal ball and I cannot predict the future. Parenthetically, two of my patients have given me the gift of a crystal ball (where the heck do you buy those?). Unfortunately, both are malfunctioning and have not provided me a glimpse of the future. What I do tell patients is that I am committed and available to provide care for them in the future regardless of what occurs. When performing surgical removal of malignant disease, the term surgeons use is *operation with curative intent*. Currently, the problem surgical oncologists face is the inability to detect subclinical or microscopic foci of cancer (though many of us are working on this limitation). So we remove all of the detectable cancer, realizing malicious malignant cells may be hiding elsewhere in the patient's body, waiting to arise in the imponderable future.

In general, conversations related to a major decision about proceeding with an operation on the liver, pancreas, colon, lungs, or wherever the cancer is located are short. Nevertheless, I have learned that patients and their families do hear what is said. Perhaps this is because I reiterate key points several times and I ask them to give me feedback indicating they understand. This is particularly important for those patients who do develop a problem or a complication after an operation. Whether it's an infection in their abdominal incision requiring antibiotics or opening the incision, or a major issue like liver insufficiency or a life-threatening pneumonia, when I discuss the treatment of the problem, patients and their families generally acknowledge that they were aware these complications might occur. Still, it is a difficult situation for the patient, concerned family members and friends, and the treating surgeon. No surgeon wants a patient to suffer any ill effects caused by the surgeon's action. We are tightrope walkers performing procedures designed to rid the patient of malignant disease. We know there is always a risk of slipping and falling from the high wire and suffering an undesirable outcome.

As I mentioned, there are caveats and disclaimers. I recognize most patients referred to me have already been thinking about surgical treatment. They have considered their options, had an operation recommended by their primary physician or medical oncologist, and are emotionally prepared to accept an aggressive therapeutic procedure. Cancer patients want the malignant tumors removed when data supports the operation and it can be performed with an acceptable probability of a safe and successful result. Acceptable probability is difficult to define; research has demonstrated cancer patients are often willing to undergo invasive or toxic treatments more readily than the physicians providing the treatment would recommend. Patients will accept the risks and pain connected with an oncological surgical procedure when there is an opportunity to eliminate their cancer. A tacit understanding exists between patient and surgeon recognizing that although complications might arise, the potential benefits outweigh the alternative of a cancer-related death.

I am compelled to reiterate an important point: Patients generally respect their physicians and recognize the hard work and years of training needed to develop their expertise and excellence.

The level of trust granted to me as a surgeon is immense. I occasionally forget that the surgical acts I perform routinely are a source of amazement to patients, medically naïve individuals, or young acolytes like our medical students. Commonly I will ask a surgical fellow, resident, or medical student who scrubbed into an operation with me what they thought about the procedure. The usual response is an expression of surprise or astonishment. That makes me happy because I can use the emotion of the moment to teach a vital lesson: the respect and trust we are granted as physicians by our patients is a precious gift to be cherished and nurtured. Patients and their families and friends are awed by the procedures my colleagues and I can perform; I am awed by their belief and confidence in us.

Humans consider odds and risk-benefit ratios many times every day, albeit not always consciously. Can I make it through that yellow light before it turns red? Can I hustle across the street before that car comes through? This operation has a chance of ridding me of my cancer.

Go for it.

15
Good Morning!

"Balance, peace, and joy are the fruit of a successful life. It starts with recognizing your talents and finding ways to serve others by using them."

Thomas Kinkade

Joyfulness: Feeling, expressing, or causing great pleasure and happiness

Early one morning last week my cell phone dinged notifying me of a new text message. This happens twenty or thirty times daily as I receive reports or questions from surgical residents, my secretary, patients, friends, or home. I opened the message and a smile quickly spread across my face.

Hi Dr. Curley. Today is the 9th anniversary of my Whipple operation. I'm still here! Thank you.

What a nice start to my frenetic day!
My grin was gradually replaced by a wistful expression.

Pancreatic adenocarcinoma, also known as pancreatic ductal adenocarcinoma (PDAC), is one of the most lethal diseases we tangle with in oncology. Epidemiologists estimate there were approximately 54,000 new cases of pancreatic adenocarcinoma diagnosed in the United States in 2017. Of greater concern is the prediction that by 2030 there will be approximately 80,000 new cases annually. More than 41,000 Americans will die from PDAC this year; it is the fourth most common cause of cancer death in women (after lung, breast, and colorectal cancer) and in men (after lung, prostate, and colorectal cancer). The long-term survival probabilities are daunting. In most countries, fewer than 5 percent of patients with PDAC will still be alive five years after their diagnosis.

PDAC is particularly deadly for several reasons. A key driver mutation in the development and propagation of PDAC is an alteration in the KRAS gene (KRAS encodes for a protein involved in cell-signaling pathways that control cell growth, cell maturation, and cell death. Mutated forms of the KRAS gene may cause cancer cells to grow and spread in the body). Cancer clinicians have not yet been able to do much with this information to help identify, detect, and treat patients at risk of developing PDAC, which may be present for years, growing insidiously in an unsuspecting and asymptomatic patient, before it becomes clinically evident.

If located in the head or uncinate process of the pancreas, these cancers are most frequently diagnosed when they obstruct the bile duct coursing from the liver through the head of the pancreas to drain into the small intestine. Patients will develop jaundice. Patients with tumors situated in the body or tail of the pancreas may present with mild or moderate abdominal or back pain, changes in gastrointestinal functions manifest as bloating or reduced appetite, or unexplained and unplanned weight loss.

Sadly, by the time the majority of patients develop these symptoms, to quote my grandmother, "The mare is out of the barn." Most patients diagnosed with PDAC have advanced-stage disease. This means that either the primary pancreatic cancer has grown around critical blood vessels like the superior mesenteric artery, or has already metastasized to lymph nodes and other organs like the liver. Metastasis from PDAC is usually a harbinger of doom. PDAC is notoriously difficult to treat and modern chemotherapy or radiation only buys a few additional months of life for patients. Once this malignant serpent slithers out, making its presence known, it rapidly invades other areas and organs and evades attempts to push it back into a hole.

The only patients who have an opportunity for prolonged survival after detection of this malicious disease are those with a reasonably small tumor that has not metastasized and can be removed with a surgical operation. This select group considered for surgical resection comprises fewer than 20 percent of PDAC patients. This grim reality becomes even harsher, because about three-quarters of these surgically treated patients develop recurrent PDAC from the microscopic metastatic deposits that are present, but undetectable at the time of their operation. I have several hundred patients with primary or metastatic liver cancers who have survived more than five and, in many cases, more than ten years after their surgical procedures. I can count on both of my hands without using all of the fingers the number of patients who are ten-year survivors after resection of PDAC.

The Whipple operation my patient mentioned in her text message has a long name in Doc Talk: a pancreaticoduodenectomy. How's that for a medical mouthful? A word worthy of a spelling bee champion. Designed to remove cancers in the head or uncinate process of the pancreas, this procedure is one of the most challenging in gastrointestinal surgical oncology. The operation removes the head of the pancreas, the entire first portion of the intestine, called the duodenum, the last one third of the stomach that connects to the duodenum (unless the surgeon chooses an option called a pylorus-sparing procedure), the first few inches of the second part of the small intestine, the gallbladder, and a portion of the bile duct above the duodenum and the head of the pancreas. After all of these structures are removed, there are three surgical reconnections that must be performed. The remaining pancreas must be attached to the small intestine to allow pancreatic enzymes needed for normal digestion of food to drain into the intestine. Next, the bile duct must be attached to the small intestine to allow normal flow of bile from the liver to enter the intestine. Finally, the stomach itself must be reconnected to the intestine to allow food to pass into the small intestine for digestion into basic protein, carbohydrate, and fat molecules that are absorbed across the lining of the small bowel, and then fed up to the liver through the portal vein to allow processing and distribution. It all sounds like a delivery, sorting, warehousing, and redistribution enterprise.

This operation has long been considered a surgical tour de force. It is a complex procedure, which in the hands of experienced hepatopancreaticobiliary, or HPB (are we running out of letters yet?), surgeons, can last from four to ten hours. Similar to any operation of long duration and multiple steps, intraoperative and postprocedure complications can and will develop. It is common for cancers in this location to abut or even invade the portal vein. It was once thought that portal-vein incursion by PDAC was a contraindication to resection, but aggressive surgical groups worldwide have demonstrated that the portal vein can be removed and replaced with a vein graft from elsewhere in the body. The short- and long-term outcomes for patients undergoing vascular reconstruction are similar to PDAC patients without portal-venous involvement.

The greater problem is tumor involvement of the superior mesenteric artery. This critical vessel supplies the arterial blood flow to the entire small intestine and more than half of the colon. Unlike blood vessels in other areas of the body, medical science has not yet devised a surefire way to replace this blood vessel. Therefore, even with no evidence of metastatic disease, pancreatic cancer that abuts or encases this artery is labeled "locally advanced" and is considered unresectable—or borderline resectable, in the event the tumor shrinks away from the vessel with preoperative chemotherapy or chemoradiation treatment.

To the great frustration of oncology professionals, only a small fraction of patients are considered candidates for resection for pancreatic adenocarcinoma. Most patients already have advanced or metastatic disease at the time of diagnosis, so they are treated with various chemotherapy recipes or combinations of chemotherapy and radiation therapy in attempts to slow the growth of the cancer. Radiation therapy can assist in alleviating some of the pain caused when the cancer begins to grow into nerves in front of the spine. State-of-the-art chemotherapy drugs improve the average survival time by only a matter of months, however. A new drug was approved for general use in PDAC patients in 2016; it improved average survival rates by a whopping two months (almost). And chemotherapy or radiation therapy is not curative in patients with PDAC. This is a source of incredible angst and exasperation for patients, their families, and their physicians.

Researchers worldwide are actively looking for better and less toxic treatments for PDAC and other cancers. Currently, immunotherapy holds tremendous promise in the treatment of numerous types of cancer. There are many clinical trials using activated

T-cells (circulating cells from the immune system) and agents that promote killing of cancer by these T-cells. The trials are still in their infancy and it remains to be seen if this latest set of promising agents coupled with cancer-killing T-cells will improve the long-term survival probability of patients with PDAC and other heinous malignant diseases.

My laboratory is actively engaged in novel, noninvasive electromagnetic-field therapies to treat PDAC. We have information in pancreatic cancer cells and in animals with PDAC indicating these electromagnetic-field treatments, which are nontoxic and harmless to normal tissues and organs, can alter the cancer cells themselves. This makes them more susceptible to killing by cytotoxic drugs, and can enhance blood flow into the tumor, increasing the delivery of anticancer drugs, nanoparticles, and activated immune cells. It is probable that this treatment will also enhance the killing of PDAC cells by standard ionizing irradiation, but the overarching goal in our laboratory is to develop less toxic therapies to improve the outcomes in our patients. We have not treated any human patients yet, but we are gaining important insights into how to use noninvasive electromagnetic fields to improve several types of treatment in cancer patients.

I mused about the fear a diagnosis of PDAC incites in patients and their family members after I received the heartwarming text from my patient. I believe she has a very high probability of becoming a ten-year survivor. It has not been an easy road for her, however. During the nine years after her operation she endured four hospitalizations for a condition called ascending cholangitis: bacteria from her intestine colonized her bile ducts and caused a life-threatening infection. During two of these hospital admissions she wound up in the intensive-care unit for more than a week with high fevers, and she actually required a ventilator for several days during one of the episodes. Each time aggressive medical therapy and antibiotics brought her back from the brink. She also required two additional operations for small-bowel obstructions. Patients who undergo major abdominal operations are known to have an increased risk of developing scarring within the peritoneal cavity, which can lead to narrowing or obstruction of the intestine. Some of these patients can be managed without an operation, and their bowel function returns to normal. My "Nine-Year Lady" unfortunately twice developed complete obstruction of her small bowel, three years and then again seven years after her initial pancreaticoduodenectomy, necessitating operations to remove a small section of scarred intestine that was in danger of perforating. Despite these problems, thankfully, her PDAC has never recurred.

My patient is one of the most grateful and radiant individuals I have encountered in my medical career. Throughout her recurrent hospitalizations and recovery she has remained upbeat and positive. She is mischievous and energetic; every time I see her in the clinic I am guaranteed a hug and kiss. She likes bright-red lipstick so the clinic staff must always quietly remind me to wipe my cheek after I see her lest I bounce into another patient's examination room with, literally, one rosy, red cheek!

I despise this hideous, difficult-to-treat disease, and I deplore what it does to the lives of far too many patients and their families. My colleagues and I are fueled by this negative emotion to search tirelessly for improved treatments for PDAC. This can be said about any type of cancer, or for that matter any type of disease a physician focuses on in his or her practice and research. It is our desire to improve not only survival but also the quality of life for our patients. That is the "driver mutation" in the genome of a physician-investigator. When it comes to PDAC, I hope someday it will not be quite so unusual to receive a text message celebrating long-term success. Such a message is a great start to a day. I texted my reply:

Good morning to you! You are welcome!

I want many more good mornings for patients.

16

The Wrestler

"Remember you will not always win. Some days, the most resourceful individual will taste defeat. But there is, in this case, always tomorrow—after you have done your best to achieve success today."

Maxwell Maltz

Resourcefulness: The ability to find quick and clever ways to overcome difficulties

I have fond memories of both of my grandfathers from when I was a boy growing up in the American Southwest. My mother's father was a master gardener. In an arid environment he was able to grow plants that should have thrived only in tropical rain forests. Botanists from the Department of Biology at the local university surveyed his garden, and promptly asked him to help with problems they were experiencing in their greenhouses. There were large fruit trees scattered throughout my grandfather's backyard, perfect for climbing and eating apples, peaches, or cherries fresh off the branch. Their dense foliage made it possible to hide and pounce down on unsuspecting younger brothers or cousins wandering too near the danger zone. Not saying I ever did such a thing, just saying it was possible. You know?

Every Friday night members of our extended family ate dinner at my mother's parents' house. I poignantly remember an after-dinner ritual. My grandfather would retire to his recliner, tooth-pick in his mouth, and instruct one of his grandchildren to turn on the color television in the bulky, multicomponent–console, with built-in radio, turntable, and speakers. It was time to watch Friday-night boxing. There was no remote control; we kids were the channel changers and volume-knob manipulators. My grand-father was usually not an emotional man, but he would become quite animated and occasionally agitated watching a fight, par-ticularly if there was a boxer he favored in the match. We grand-children enjoyed watching him more than we did the pugilists on the flickering television screen.

My father's father, on the other hand, was a wrestling fan. By wrestling, I mean the brawling seen on Saturday-afternoon televi-sion, featuring men in tight shorts and outlandish costumes, some wearing colorful capes and hoods or masks over their heads. They entered the ring to either wild applause or catcalls and hisses, bouncing off the ropes to clothesline their onrushing opponent or jumping from the turnbuckles to land on their hapless rival laid out on the mat below. Even to a boy it was obviously bad theater and fraud, but I enjoyed watching my grandfather yelling at the television, berating the bad guys and the referees. He knew every hero and villain, and he would hurl epithets at the masked men in tight wrestling suits while openly cheering for those he admired. I still remember some of their names. Gene Kiniski, The Sheik, Ray Mendoza, Dory Funk Jr., Terry Funk, Mad Dog Vachon, Hard Boiled Haggarty, Raul Reyes, Killer Kowalski, and Johnny Valentine. My grandfather particularly loved the chaos of tag-team matches, guaranteed to degenerate into a free-for-all with all the combatants in the ring, throwing chairs, and occasionally even body-slamming the referee to the canvas. When I grew older I mistakenly pointed out that these matches were all rehearsed and the outcomes were scripted, that this wasn't real sport. He fixed me with a glare and informed me I was getting, "a little too big for my britches." He asked me if I thought a 250-pound man climbing to the top of the ropes to hurl himself on his foe below, or the prostrate, seemingly stunned wrestler on the mat absorbing the flying blow should be considered as anything less than athletic.

Good point. I wouldn't want to do it.

Cancer patients and caregivers grapple with malignant disease every day. Surgical oncology is an unusual, but not unique, subspecialty area in surgical care. Many surgeons will enter the lives of their patients for an acute illness or event, perform the indicated operation to improve their condition, care for them in the hospital, and then see them for one or two postoperative visits before discharging them on to the rest of their lives. Some surgical subspecialties, including surgical oncology, follow their patients longitudinally. All oncology-related specialties follow their patients for years, if not their lifetime, after a diagnosis of cancer. We watch for the success of our treatment, evidence of any recurrent or new metastatic disease, and we treat any symptoms or problems related to the therapies we deliver. We get a chance to know our patients and their families, and to watch how they respond to living with the ever-present specter—the possible return of malignant disease.

I admire the pluck and defiance of my patients who have a never-give-up attitude. One particular patient comes to mind when I think about fortitude. When I walked into the examination room to meet him, he sprang to his feet, grasped my hand

and shook it vigorously, smiled a dazzling white smile, and then gave me a bear hug. Effusive. His first words: "Doc, you're going to help me beat this thing!" At this point he was still shaking my hand, his grip getting tighter, so I politely asked him to release my hand lest I be unable to perform an operation on him because of damaged digits. He laughed and immediately cut me loose, allowing circulation to return to my fingers. We sat down to talk. I was not surprised this gentleman had an impressive grip. He was in his late forties and built like a running back or rugby player. I actually asked him if he had been a football player. He feigned disgust and exasperation and said, "No, I'm a real athlete. I am a wrestler." As I explored his history it turned out he had been a collegiate wrestler of significant accomplishment and repute. After graduation he had founded a successful business and spent his time raising his family, expanding his business acumen, and refereeing high school and college wrestling matches around his home state.

I was seeing this man for a diagnosis of colorectal-cancer liver metastasis. Eight months prior to our initial meeting, he noticed some blood in his bowel movements and made an appointment with his primary-care physician. His doctor noted that he did have blood on a rectal exam and that he was slightly anemic. The patient had no family history of colon cancer. A gastroenterologist was consulted and a colonoscopy revealed a colon cancer. The patient underwent an operation in his hometown to remove the malignant colon tumor. Pathology revealed cancer in several lymph nodes near the primary tumor, and a biopsy of a liver tumor confirmed metastasis in the right lobe of his liver. He had stage IV disease, signifying blood-borne spread of malignant cells with successful implantation and growth of cells from the colon cancer to another organ, his liver.

The patient recovered from his colon operation at a "meteoric pace" (according to his hometown surgeon when I spoke to him), and then received six months of systemic intravenous chemotherapy. He was referred to me to address the sole clinically evident site of malignant disease, the tumor in the right lobe of his liver. I use the phrase *clinically evident* purposefully; the radiologists and I did not detect any suspicious tumors or lesions in his lungs, lymph nodes, or peritoneal cavity on our state-of-the-art CT scans. This remarkably fit, healthy young man had just a solitary liver metastasis smack-dab in the middle of the right lobe. An almost Pavlovian circumstance for a hepatobiliary surgical oncologist who loves to attack and remove liver malignancies.

This gentleman was one of the most energetic, positive, let's-get-this-done people I have met—in any area of my life. We talked for about half an hour during our first visit, and I completed a physical examination. I reviewed his CT scans and pathology information; he had a five-centimeter liver tumor, which was originally almost eight centimeters in diameter. The reduction indicated a positive response to chemotherapy. Numerous studies have indicated that patients showing shrinkage of their tumors with chemotherapy tend to have a longer survival time after surgical and other anticancer therapies. But, as I've said, it's all statistics and probabilities; the bottom line is we can never know what's going to happen specifically to any one patient. The wrestler told me he was ready for me to operate and "get this devil out of me" as quickly as possible. The next week I performed an exploratory laparotomy.

Surgeons are multisensory creatures. We like to visually inspect the area of operation, but we also like to feel. I palpated my patient's lymph nodes near the blood vessels heading into his liver. Several of them felt hard like small stones, but not enlarged. I removed all of these regional lymph nodes and then completed a routine right hepatectomy. Upon checking the remainder of the belly cavity visually and tactilely, there was no evidence of tumor at any other site.

My patient was up walking laps in the hallways of the surgical unit the night of his operation. Several nurses told me they were exhausted just watching him. He was indefatigable. He consistently had a huge smile on his face and greeted everyone with a bone-crushing handshake. He left the hospital only four days after his operation. As he stated, "All systems are working, I'm outta here."

See ya!

I saw him in the clinic the following week and we reviewed the results from the surgery. I explained that the pathologist had found not only the single liver tumor we knew was present, but also three additional two-to-three-millimeter tumors near it. None of these tumors were close to the liver transection line, meaning we had achieved a negative-margin operation. Furthermore, three of the twelve lymph nodes removed from around the blood vessels supplying his liver contained metastatic colorectal cancer.

He was nonplussed, and asked if it was still possible to be cured, the question I get every week from many of my patients. I explained the finding of the small tumors in the liver combined with lymph-node metastases meant there was a high probability he could have microscopic cancer cells hiding elsewhere in his body. In other words, his chance for long-term cancer-free survival was significantly reduced, but it was not zero. I finished with the assurance that I planned to follow him closely and watch for any recurrence. That earned me a grand smile, more damage to my right hand, and an exhalation-inducing embrace.

He returned home and spoke to his medical oncologist. They decided to proceed with another six months of a different chemotherapy regimen. At the end of the second six months of cytotoxic drugs, he returned to see me in the clinic. All of his blood tests and CT scans showed no problem, no clinically evident cancer.

I wasn't sure if my right hand or my chest was going to remain intact thanks to this patient.

Unfortunately, the good results and good news were short lived. Six months later, a blood test we measure in patients with colorectal cancer called carcinoembryonic antigen (CEA), was elevated in him. When I saw his lab results, I immediately scrolled through his CT scans, and then quietly cursed at the computer screen. He had four new tumors in the hypertrophied left lobe of his liver along with at least a dozen small lung metastases scattered throughout both lungs.

I walked into the examination room to tell him the news. He knew from my face I was about to drop a bomb on him. Before I could say anything, he stood up, hugged me, and to my amazement said, "We'll beat this thing!" I reassured him we were in the fight together and then I went over all of his results. He sat, quietly nodding and occasionally asking for clarification. Finally he asked, "Okay, what's our next move?" I spoke with my colleagues in medical oncology, and we determined a new sequence of drugs to treat him for this rapid recurrence.

At a visit with me three months later, he launched the question patients often ask, he wanted to know how long he would live. He was a motivated, insightful, intelligent individual, and as we sat together in a clinic room, he rifled through copies of scientific papers describing chemotherapy and novel treatments for stage IV colorectal cancer. He noted from his reading the median survival rate with the chemotherapy drugs he was receiving ranged from eighteen to twenty-four months. I affirmed that those perceptions and statistics were correct, but there was no way to predict if he would live less or more time than the average. He laughed, tossed the research papers on the floor, and said, "These don't describe me!"

This man was tough. He kept working despite major surgical procedures and significant side effects from chemotherapy. He was also a fountain of optimism, regardless of seemingly daunting odds against him. He found a way to make things work. I certainly was not going to shoot holes in his belief he was going to beat the odds and outlive the predictions.

After six months of additional chemotherapy, CT scans of this gentleman's chest showed the lung metastases had completely disappeared, and the liver metastases appeared to be calcified scar tissue. His CEA blood test had returned to a normal value. After considering his situation and excellent antitumor response in a tumor-board meeting, my colleagues and I decided we would stop chemotherapy and follow him. This we did with blood tests, CT scans, and physical examinations every three months for another year.

At the one-year mark, his CEA value was again elevated and CT scans revealed recurrence in the liver, lungs, and peritoneal cavity. Grimly, I walked into the examination room to have a heartrending discussion. As I reviewed the test results, his wife quietly wept. Before addressing me, he turned to her, gave her a hug, and told her he would be all right. He pivoted to me, flashed a dazzling smile, and said, "Remember, we are in this together."

Yes, we are.

Based on probabilities, patterns, and the rapid recurrence of his cancer in multiple sites, this man would have been predicted to survive no more than two or three years after his initial cancer diagnosis. Recently I received a note from his brother informing me my patient had finally lost the battle (his brother's words) and had passed away—almost eight years after his original cancer diagnosis. Throughout those years I saw him every three months and arranged for him to meet numerous specialists administering a variety of new clinical trials for colorectal cancer. His medical oncologist at home was, and still is, very active in treating patients with established and new regimens for gastrointestinal malignancies. Whenever we spoke on the phone about our mutual patient, it was always with a note of admiration for his courage and formidable spirit.

I loved watching boxers and faux wrestlers (performance athletes?) with my grandfathers. Several of the wrestlers we saw on Saturday-afternoon television had been college wrestlers, some even competing in the Olympics. They were indeed athletes. Not great actors, but athletes nonetheless. Perhaps the ability to work hard, to strive, to endure pain and discomfort and defeat is what led my patient, the wrestler, to survive as long as he did. I have seen similar powerful and courageous efforts from patients of all ages and backgrounds. I am reminded of words from one of my favorite songs, "The Boxer," performed by Paul Simon and Art Garfunkel describing a fighter who is cut, knocked down, and beaten in the ring, but he chooses to remain and battle on.

Warrior terminology abounds in the cancer lexicon: "The war on cancer." "She lost her battle with cancer." "I am fighting cancer." "We are going to attack your cancer with every weapon in our arsenal." "He refuses to surrender and will keep battling." "She is soldiering on through this fight with cancer." "I am going to beat and defeat this cancer." "It was a courageous fight." "We have your cancer on the ropes."

Patients diagnosed with cancer and treated with our multidisciplinary approaches are knocked down physically and emotionally, but they pick themselves up off the canvas and struggle on. They carry the reminders of the acute and chronic side effects from cytotoxic chemotherapy and radiation-induced skin and functional-organ changes. They endure the scars, complications, and impairments imposed by the blades of surgical oncologists like me. Though sometimes they want to, they don't leave. They remain. They maintain. I respect the effort, the invincible spirit, and the patients who don't give a damn about the odds or probabilities; they are going out swinging. We are tag-team partners in oncology, entering the ring to attack cancer with every move and method we know. Hell, I'll even throw a few chairs if it will help.

Indomitable. The wrestler.

Respect, my brother.

17

The Deacon's Wife
aka "The Real Muhthuh"

"Faith consists of believing when it is beyond the power of reason to believe."

Voltaire

Faith: *Complete trust or confidence in someone or something*

We surgeons would not be able to perform major operations safely without the collaboration and cooperation of our anesthesiology colleagues. Hepatobiliary surgeons ask their friendly neighborhood anesthesiologist to maintain low central-venous pressure (CVP) anesthesia during liver resections. This means the patient is maintained in a slightly dehydrated state to reduce the pressure in the vena cava, and as a result, in the hepatic veins that drain directly into the vena cava near the heart. Bleeding caused by high CVP, in the range of four-to-ten millimeters of mercury of pressure, transmitted back into the hepatic veins coursing through the liver is a bane of the existence of the liver resectionist. We can easily control the blood vessels (specifically the portal vein and hepatic-arterial branches) flowing *into* the area of the liver being removed. But bleeding from unintentional avulsion of small branches or minor rents in the thin-walled, fragile hepatic veins draining blood *out* of the liver can increase intra-operative blood loss. Though preventable, this is potentially problematic, higher volumes of bleeding will occur unless low CVP is maintained. Most hepatobiliary surgeons prefer to keep the CVP as low as possible, from negative one to one millimeter of mercury if the patient's blood pressure, heart rate, and kidney function are stable at these low pressures.

Oncological surgeons are fastidious about avoiding blood loss because we prefer that our patients not require or receive transfusions. We are not concerned about style points, but we limit blood loss because, while controversial, multiple clinical studies over the past two decades suggest blood transfusions during or shortly after cancer surgery inhibit components of the immune system and increase the likelihood of recurrence of malignant disease, reducing the patient's probability of long-term survival. This is a frequent "Current Controversies" discussion in national and international surgical oncology meetings. Currently, for some types of cancer, evidence suggests a causative relationship between blood transfusion and a higher risk of cancer recurrence, and more rapid cancer recurrence. So the question has been raised often and is definitely on the radar of the surgical oncologist. Thus, during an operation, close communication and ongoing conversation with our anesthesia colleagues "on the other side of the drape" is mandatory to optimize intra-operative care, reduce blood loss, and maximize patient safety.

After a routine scheduled operation is completed, the patient is transported to the recovery room, also called the Post-Anesthesia Care Unit, or PACU. Patients generally remain in the PACU for a few hours to allow nurses to closely monitor their vital signs and to assure they are recovering well from the effects of anesthesia. General anesthesia and narcotic pain medications often used directly after major surgical procedures combine to produce some interesting reactions in patients. Dissociative events are common, meaning the patient, while obviously a bit groggy, is apparently awake and able to converse and respond to questions. Occasionally, people in this early postanesthetic state will blurt out bizarre, nonsensical, unexpected, or inappropriate remarks. Interestingly, the person usually has no recollection of the comments. This phenomenon has led intelligence services worldwide to use anesthetic drugs, like the barbiturate sodium pentothal, as a "truth serum." Great material for spy novels and movies, but the truth is there's no predicting what somebody may say after receiving a dose of psychoactive anesthetic drugs.

Some years ago, an almost-seventy-year-old woman was referred to me after being diagnosed with a rare hepatic tumor, epithelioid hemangioendothelioma. EHE is an interesting tumor that can present as solitary or multiple lesions within the liver, and it can arise in other organs as well. EHE originating in the liver is scarce indeed; only several dozen are diagnosed annually in the United States. Not all EHEs are malignant; some have little or no propensity to spread elsewhere. But the lungs are the most common site for metastasis from malignant EHE in the liver. Malignant EHE is biologically fascinating because there are documented episodes of removal of the liver tumors that led to reduction or even resolution of lung metastases in some patients. When local treatment (like surgical removal or ionizing-radiation therapy) of a tumor at one site in the body leads to reduction in the size of metastatic lesions in other organs like this, it is known as the abscopal effect. In oncology, we wish we witnessed abscopal events more frequently. Unfortunately, like EHE, it is relatively rare.

My new patient was diagnosed with EHE when routine blood

tests during her annual physical examination revealed mild inflammation of the liver. Her family practitioner thought this might be related to gallstones so an ultrasound study was performed. It showed a normal gallbladder but also detected a six-centimeter tumor in the left lobe of her liver. After a CT scan and needle biopsies of the tumor were obtained, she was referred to me to consider surgical management.

This woman was a quiet, prim, proper, and reserved individual. She was accompanied to her first office visit by her husband and three adult daughters. They were from a small town in east Texas, and when I asked them questions, their most frequent response was a simple "Yes, Sir" or "No, Sir." The patient's husband was a businessman in their community, and felt it was important to inform me that he was a deacon at the local Baptist church, where his wife and daughters were also Sunday school teachers. After my patient's children were grown and had left the house, she worked as a secretary at the church. Prior to being diagnosed with epithelioid hemangioendothelioma, the patient had been in good overall health, having only mild hypertension that was well controlled with a single medication. She was active, engaged in her church and community activities, and proud of her children and grandchildren. She told me she was not worried about undergoing an operation because she knew she was going to be well.

This woman and her family were salt-of-the-earth folks.

A couple of weeks after meeting this calm, unpretentious lady, I performed a straightforward surgery to remove the tumor-bearing left lobe of her liver. The operation took approximately one hour to perform; it was routine, unremarkable, and uncomplicated, and she was completely stable throughout. Her blood loss was minimal and transfusion was never considered or necessary. I walked out to the family waiting room and informed my patient's husband and daughters that the operation had gone well and she was stable and resting comfortably in the PACU. When they asked to see her, I said they could go to the PACU in one hour. I mentioned that by then she should be awake enough to talk with them.

Fate occasionally intervenes at opportune moments. By sheer coincidence, a surgical oncology fellow who was born and bred in the borough of Brooklyn in New York and had the accent and attitude to prove it, was on my service that day. He and I went to check on our patient in the PACU at the same moment her husband and three daughters arrived at her bedside. Before I could say anything, her husband grasped her hand and asked with concern, "How are you, Honey?"

From her mouth erupted a string of invectives, curses, words banned for on-air use by the Federal Communication Commission, and open questions about the parentage, lineage, and even species of every person present. Her husband recoiled a few steps and grasped his chest, asking, "Honey, are you all right?"

Almost seventy years of suppressed foul language again poured forth from this respectable church lady. One of her daughters managed to utter a monosyllabic question, "Mom?" More cursing. Swear words used as nouns, verbs, adjectives, and adverbs; it was a masterful extravaganza of expletives.

Four astonished family members turned to me, and one asked, "Is this normal?"

No. No it is not. But it happens.

In a state of psychic shock, one of the daughters said, "She is not acting like my mother."

At that moment, my fellow, apparently caught up in the dissociative frenzy, muttered audibly, "Oh, she's a real Muhthuh, all right!" The Brooklyn accent was icing on the cake.

There was a pause of stunned silence. Suddenly, all three of my patient's daughters started laughing. Loud, hold-on-to-your-belly, tears-running-down-your-cheeks guffaws.

The fellow apologized, "Uh, sorry 'bout dat comment," causing them to laugh louder. We were creating quite a scene in the PACU. I wanted to laugh because of the absurdity and improbability of what had just transpired, but I refrained, fearing the husband's blasphemy-induced angina pectoris (he was still clutching his chest) would be converted to a full-blown myocardial infarction if I chuckled openly.

Primum non nocere (First, do no harm), right?

During our riotous commotion, the patient had drifted back into postanesthetic sleep. Staring at his wife in disbelief, my patient's husband shook his head and mustered a weak smile. Clearly incredulous about what he had just heard, he told me he needed to go sit down for a few minutes. His daughters pulled it together, and I escorted them out of the PACU. As we walked I explained that anesthetic agents and pain medications may sometimes cause unusual comments and behaviors in patients. I admitted I had never heard anything quite like that explosive, profane tirade, but I reassured them this was not a lasting side effect of the operation or the anesthesia. One of the daughters pulled me aside and exclaimed, "I didn't think she even knew all of those words!"

Now she knew.

I quietly returned to the PACU and stood at the end of my snoring patient's bed. I hoped I was correct and the profligate profusion of profanity was a drug-induced, solitary, and never-to-be-repeated episode. A PACU nurse strolled by and simply said, "Wow!"

Yeah, wow!

The next morning my fellow and I visited the patient in her hospital room. Her husband and three daughters sat expectantly awaiting our arrival. Again, before I could say anything, one of the daughters spoke, "Tell her. Tell her what she said yesterday."

My patient looked at me with pleading eyes, "Please tell me I didn't say anything rude or inappropriate?"

Well, Ma'am, I can't exactly do that. Clearly, the patient's husband and daughters had told her about the profundity of profanity she had loosed upon us after her operation. I didn't recount the details, but I did confirm she had used some words that would have gotten my mouth washed out with soap had I said them as a boy. She blushed furiously and apologized to her family, my fellow, and me. Her daughters and husband (now fully in the spirit of the ridiculous) started laughing, and one of the daughters pointed to my fellow and said, "He has a great name for you, Mom. A real Muhthuh!" We all laughed.

Well, not all. My horrified patient continued to blush and apologize.

I can happily report that the church lady recovered uneventfully from her operation. Her EHE never recurred or metastasized to another site, despite having malignant features like vascular invasion. I never again heard her emit a word that would earn an R rating at a movie theater. Nonetheless, her husband and daughters were relentless and ruthless every time I saw her in the clinic. At each visit, when I first entered the examination room, one of them would exclaim, "The real Muhthuh is here to see you!" The poor lady would simply blush and apologize at least half a dozen times. I couldn't convince any of them to let it go, it had become family lore. Parenthetically, the three daughters with slow, east Texas drawls all developed good imitations of a Brooklyn accent.

Later that year, in December, my patient had a scheduled appointment with me in the clinic. She presented me with a wrapped box and sheepishly stated, "This is to make up for the nasty things I said to you."

I smiled and reassured her a gift was not necessary. I promised her I was not offended. I'm a surgeon, after all. She insisted I open the box. My patients frequently have talents I know nothing about unless I follow them over time and learn about their skills, hobbies, and aptitudes. Inside the box was a beautiful wooden Santa Claus. It was a single, solid piece of wood and on the surface my patient had painted a face, features, arms, and a sack full of gifts. It seemed as though the wood had been shaped perfectly for the exceptional object of art. She asked me if I recognized the wood. I confessed I did not. Sitting beside her, her husband proudly informed me it was a cypress knee. Cypress knees arise from the underwater or underground roots of cypress trees that grow in swamps or boggy soil. My patient would venture out to the wild cypress groves near her home a few times every year to select and harvest a collection of cypress knees. She would study the shape of the wood to discern the character hidden within, polish the wood, and then paint intricate faces and features onto each piece. She had no formal art training. Remarkable. Every figure was unique. A spectacular specimen of homemade art destined to become a prized family heirloom. I thanked her for the exquisite gift.

She smiled, and apologized again.

The next December, she presented me with a second box. Inside was another cypress-knee Santa Claus. It was amazing and very different from the previous year's Kris Kringle, but equally beautiful. Recognizing a developing trend, I thanked her repeatedly, but I asked her to not give me any more of these heartfelt gifts. I appreciated her efforts, gratitude, and talent, and I told her I would prefer that she gave these to other people. She informed me that she gave her cypress-knee figures to friends and family members, and sometimes sold them at craft fairs and donated the money to a local shelter for the homeless. A good-hearted woman, I was touched by her thoughtfulness.

The deacon's wife lived for more than a decade after I removed the unusual liver cancer. Toward the end of her life, she developed Alzheimer's disease and stopped coming for annual visits. But while I was still seeing her routinely, she could not escape the good-natured teasing from her husband and daughters. They refused to forget "the time Momma cussed out us and Dr. Curley." When she passed away, her daughters sent a note thanking me for my care and for the additional years they, and their children, had gotten to spend with this extraordinary woman.

I still have the cypress-knee Santa Claus figures. They are carefully wrapped and stored each year to be displayed on my mantel during the Christmas season. Every time I unpack them, I smile remembering the story of "the real Muhthuh."

Why the @%&# wouldn't I?

18

The Photographer

"People are like stained glass windows. They sparkle and shine when the sun is out, but when the darkness sets in, their true beauty is revealed only if there is a light from within."

Elisabeth Kübler-Ross

Beauty: A combination of qualities, such as shape, color, or form, that pleases the aesthetic senses, especially the sight

Anyone who has a cellular telephone is a photographer. People take pictures of their meals at restaurants (really?), vacations, and family, or "selfies" with pets, friends, and the occasional random minor or major celebrity they chance to encounter. I remember the days when we carried photos of our children or pets in our wallets or billfolds. Space constraints made it impossible to carry more than just a few. Now, we are not so fortunate. The seemingly endless number of pictures stored on cell phones is a dilemma.

I wish to share an opinion and an important bit of information. The coefficient of cuteness of your children, grandchildren, dog, cat, boa constrictor...whatever, drops at a logarithmic rate with the increasing number of images you feel compelled to share on your phone. The screen is small, increasing and decreasing the size of the image with your fingers is distracting, and the whole scrolling thing almost induces seizure activity. My personal limit is about three pictures. Up to that number, I am engaged and interested. I will verbally provide appropriate congratulations, sound effects ("Ooh," "Ahh," or "Nice!"), and confirm your good fortune at having a beautiful subject in the image displayed on your phone. However, after three pictures, I am finished. My excitement wanes, my eyes rapidly flick left and right seeking an escape route, and yawning is induced. This is a public-service announcement; I am not alone in these feelings about cell phone–photo overload.

In the hands and viewfinder of someone who appreciates and understands light and conditions, photography is a wonderful art form. New Mexico, where I grew up, is known for its natural effects and vivid colors in the outdoor world and man-made environments. It is not possible to visit a museum or gallery without seeing photographic scenes from around the state in color or black and white. I had two high school friends who had their own dark rooms. I was impressed by their composition, angles, and framing of photographs of different events and places. Frankly, they were not much fun when they were together, going on tediously about f-stops, light meters, and backlighting. Enough already! Hurry up and snap the picture, will you? I am smiling. This is a smile.

Obviously, I never developed an abiding interest in learning or practicing photography as an art form. Like most humans I use it indiscriminately to record family gatherings, events, or a striking sunset. I don't worry about light angles, shadows, or if the top of somebody's head is outside the frame. But I do enjoy stunning photographic images and those who capture them. One of my favorite photographers is a former patient of mine. Former, because a couple of years ago he succumbed to the cancer we battled jointly for almost a decade.

The photographer was one of those people who illuminate a room. Joy and physical presence emanated like a force field around him. When I met him in the clinic for our initial consultation, he bypassed the customary handshake and gave me a hug and a kiss on the cheek, then pulled back and said, "Great to meet you, brother!" His wife remained sitting in a chair in the examination room, and smiling she said, "What can I say? He's a happy man."

Nothing wrong with that.

Physicians are taught in medical school and in postgraduate training that cancer tends to be a disease of elderly populations. Historically, many types of malignant disease are most common in individuals in their sixties or seventies. All of us know, however, cancer can strike at any age. The photographer was an active, healthy gentleman in his mid-forties when he developed progressively worsening constipation and intermittent abdominal pain. Upon further questioning, the photographer admitted he had been feeling more fatigued than usual, but as many of us tend to do, he attributed this to a busy work schedule and getting a little older. I can't begin to count the number of times I have heard patients dismiss concerning symptoms for months or more until they are finally convinced to see a physician, only to be diagnosed with cancer. Before we met, a CT scan revealed a mass in my patient's colon, which a biopsy confirmed to be a colonic

adenocarcinoma. The scan also revealed probable liver metastases in both lobes of the liver.

The photographer was symptomatic from significant narrowing of the colonic lumen by the tumor, so a surgeon in his city
performed a routine oncological colon resection and biopsied a
liver lesion, which confirmed the presence of metastatic colon
cancer. The photographer recovered uneventfully and met with
a medical oncologist who informed him and his wife that the
finding of bilobar, multiple liver metastases was a poor prognostic
indicator—and even with chemotherapy he could expect to live
eighteen months or less. That news didn't sit well with this couple
so they referred themselves to me.

I abhor nihilistic thinking. It is correct to inform patients that
the presence of stage IV malignant disease indicates it is unlikely
they will be cured by the multidisciplinary treatments we have
available these days. Stage IV colorectal cancer in particular is
not an automatic and irrevocable death sentence. There are new
treatments and developments for many types of cancer coming
out at a remarkable pace. Furthermore, we don't "cure" patients
even of some benign diseases. Once someone is diagnosed with
diabetes, he or she will always have diabetes. The same can be
said for high blood pressure, autoimmune disorders, and neuro-
muscular derangements. But patients with these so-called benign
conditions can live long and productive lives with proper care
and treatment. There are additional variables we have no ability
to measure, predict, or control. In oncology care we occasionally
witness remarkable responses to therapy, and some patients are
able to live with their malignant disease for many years.

The photographer was not satisfied with an inevitable death
pronouncement in eighteen months. When he and his wife visited
with me and with one of my colleagues in medical oncology, we

formulated a treatment plan that included three months of chemotherapy, followed by repeat imaging with CT scans of the chest,
abdomen, and pelvis. He was a vibrant and otherwise healthy man.
He had no problems or major side effects from the chemotherapy,
and continued working at his craft throughout the cytotoxic drug
infusions.

After three months the photographer and his wife met with me
again in the clinic to discuss options and next steps. CT scans
revealed significant reduction in the size of his liver tumors,
and he had no evidence of tumors at any other site in his body. I
pointed out that the majority of his liver metastases were located
in the right hepatic lobe. There were two small, now partially
calcified (from response to the chemotherapy) tumors in his left
hepatic lobe. During our first meeting, we had already discussed
a goal of surgically removing or destroying his liver tumors, so
before I could state that I believed we were ready to proceed with
an operation he told me, "I'm ready to rock, Doc!"

That's all I needed to hear. We discussed the requisite technical details, risks, alternatives, and expectations about hospitalization and recovery time. A few weeks later I performed a right
hepatectomy, completely removing the right lobe of his liver, and
radiofrequency ablation of the scarred tumors remaining in the
left lobe of his liver. He was a thin, active gentleman so the entire
operation took less than three hours to finish. He was up walking
the following morning.

I knew from our conversations he was a professional photographer, but he had not previously shared any of his images with me.
Now that I had him as a captive audience in the hospital recovering from an operation, I asked him to show me examples of his
work.

My patient responded by pulling out a laptop computer and
placing it on the ever-present wheeled table. (You know, the

surface used for food trays, plastic water pitchers, urinals, tissues, and incentive spirometers to encourage postoperative deep breathing. I've seen thoughtful and thoughtless combinations of items on these bed tables. I apologize—a digression on tables has nothing to do with photography.) He tapped the keys of the computer for a few seconds, and a long list of files appeared. He smiled slyly, and asked, "How much time do you have, Brother?" I surveyed the file names and chose one that struck my fancy, "Music." He selected the folder icon and dozens of tiny photographic thumbnail images filled the screen. He clicked on the first one in the upper left corner and it enlarged to full size. The photographer proceeded to scroll through image after image for almost thirty minutes.

I was awestruck. More than 90 percent of the photographs were black-and-white. He confessed he preferred black-and-white because of the contrast in light, shadows, and shading he could attain using this format. The images varied from shots of bands playing on stage, close-ups of entertainers, some of whom were famous and some of whom were local artists I didn't recognize, backstage support-crew members, and the crowds and individuals enjoying the performances.

I would visit every day while he was in the hospital, and we would open another file. His work documented everything from architecture to street scenes to ordinary or important events to well-known or common people. I particularly enjoyed one series entitled simply "Shoe Shine." These images showed boys or men on the streets or in buildings around the city posing for him, or caught in the act of performing their work. The angles, the lighting, the composition, and the artistry were obvious even to me. The images drew me into a place, a moment, and a mundane but gloriously rendered and recorded service that came to life.

After recovering from his liver surgery, the photographer

received another three months of chemotherapy. We then began the nerve-racking process of routine follow-up evaluations with CT scans and blood tests, watching for any evidence of recurrence. He made it almost three years before a CT scan revealed three new liver tumors and some enlarged lymph nodes in his retroperitoneum. He resumed chemotherapy with a new regimen. After six months the lymph nodes had returned to normal size and the three liver tumors were smaller. I performed a second operation and removed two of the tumors and did radiofrequency ablation on the third. I also biopsied several of the previously enlarged lymph nodes, and was pleased to find that no malignant cells were identified by our pathologist. While the photographer was hospitalized again I used the opportunity to view more of his stunningly beautiful work.

I recognized that all of the photographs in my patient's portfolio came from the city where he and his wife lived. When I inquired about this observation, he informed me he was the official photographer for his city. I was surprised; I didn't realize cities had official photographers. It made sense and I understood why he had captured everything from buildings, street signs, street scenes, events, and people from his city.

When we reached the five-year mark after his initial cancer diagnosis, he noted sardonically that he had bypassed the eighteen-month prediction by a significant amount of time. We laughed about the grossly inaccurate forecast, and he reported he had no feelings of ill will toward the mistaken physician.

But then he suddenly developed a solemn expression. He hesitantly mentioned he had more photographs to show me, but warned they were emotionally challenging to view. His city had been severely impacted by Hurricane Katrina a few years previously. He opened a file on his laptop entitled "Hurricane" and started to scroll silently through the images. Images can speak soundlessly and evoke powerful reactions. I have no words to describe what I saw. The destruction, death, and devastation were overwhelming. He had shot photographs not only in the immediate aftermath of the storm but also for more than a year thereafter. It was gut-wrenching to view. I could only imagine how difficult it had been for the photographer to witness and record the images. His photos caught the personal expressions of pain, helplessness, and hopelessness following this catastrophic event. It was impossible not to experience a visceral reaction and at one point, I looked up as a tear was rolling down his cheek. "I can't look at these too often. It's just too much to remember."

Great photography has the ability to evoke a full range of feelings. My patient was an accomplished practitioner of his craft. He was blessed with a gift to look at common people and places and find extraordinary grace and beauty. Conversely, he was also willing to see and record pain and ugliness. He captured all aspects of life.

Almost six years after his original diagnosis, my patient's cancer recurred for the second time. He had malignant masses in the liver, lungs, and lymph nodes. Because another surgery was not an option, my colleagues concocted more chemotherapy treatments and used radiation to treat a painful area of lymph node recurrence behind his liver. Impressively, throughout all of the side effects and pain caused by his cancer and therapies, he never failed to smile when I entered his room. The invariable greeting was a hug, a kiss on the cheek, and "Hello, Brother."

The photographer continued to practice his art right up to the time he died. His images are an eternal legacy to a time, a place, and a city. He was genuine, gracious, and thankful for the common, everyday gifts he received. I learn important lessons from every patient I meet, and from every person I encounter. The lessons I learned from the photographer about noticing, observing, and enjoying fleeting, mundane events in ordinary life are indelibly etched on my soul.

Thank you to the photographer for reminding me daily to appreciate simple gifts.

19

The Rancher

"You know, you don't have to look like everybody else
to be acceptable and to feel acceptable."

Fred Rogers

*Acceptance: Agreement with or belief in an idea or
explanation; willingness to tolerate a difficult situation*

Sitting in my office I scanned the day's list of patients I was scheduled to see before walking over to the clinic. I noticed one new
patient had been diagnosed with rectal cancer. Other than the
gentleman's name and age, I had no additional information. I was
in my first month as an assistant professor of surgery after completing nine years of postgraduate training. After graduating from
medical school, the next almost-decade was divided into five years
of general-surgery residency, two years of basic science-laboratory
cancer research, and two years of surgical oncology fellowship. I
finally had what my parents called a real job. I realized the new
rectal cancer patient was scheduled to see me in ten minutes. I
ambled over to clinic.

A nurse in the clinic informed me that the patient was already in an examination room because he had arrived early. I rapped on the door and entered the room. The patient was a man in his late sixties sitting on the end of the ubiquitous, bland exam-room table. A woman, who I soon learned was his daughter, sat in a chair beside him. He was dressed in frayed but clean denim overalls; a faded, once-colorful, pearl-snap-button Western shirt; and well-worn cowboy boots. A sweat-stained straw cowboy hat lay on the adjacent desk, resting properly on the crown (never on the brim). The man was bent over at the waist and holding his chest tightly with his right hand.

Usually when I first meet a patient I shake his or her hand and introduce myself. With this gentleman my first words were a question: "How long have you been having chest pain?"

"It's been getting steadily worse for the last ten minutes," he replied. "I took a nitroglycerin tablet, but it is not letting up."

The patient's daughter informed me he had suffered a "minor heart attack" two years previously and he saw a cardiologist every few months. She reported he occasionally had chest pain when engaged in strenuous labor on their "farm," but after a few minutes of rest and sometimes a nitroglycerin tablet under his tongue, he was usually good to go. I quickly examined him. His heart rate was ninety, his skin was cool and clammy, and he was clearly having severe chest discomfort.

Crescendo angina. I had seen it once before as a surgical resident. These symptoms indicate a critical obstruction in one or more of the major coronary arteries providing blood supply to the heart. An impending, potentially lethal myocardial infarction was unfolding in the man before me. I quickly walked out the door and yelled for a nurse to call 911 and get an ambulance. A seemingly odd request given we were in a clinic building physically attached to a hospital. However, the hospital was a dedicated cancer center, well equipped to provide care for patients with all types of cancer, but definitely not a complete one-stop shopping experience for all medical care. We were certainly not prepared to handle patients with critical cardiac disease or an acute myocardial infarction.

After realizing I was serious, the nurse dialed 911 and joined me in the room. Emergency medical technicians (EMTs) were in the clinic within ten minutes. An intravenous needle was placed into the patient's arm, an oxygen cannula was inserted into his nostrils, and he was strapped into the wheeled ambulance stretcher and whisked to the nearby elevator. The patient was loaded into the ambulance idling in front of our building, and we drove, lights flashing and siren wailing, about a quarter of a mile to the emergency room of a major heart hospital across the street. I was impressed with the rapid emergency room response with blood specimens obtained, an electrocardiogram performed, and a cardiologist at his bedside within minutes. He was soon transported to the cardiac catheterization lab. Recognizing he had a higher-priority, life-threatening problem with his heart than with the rectal cancer, I asked his daughter to call and keep me informed of his status. The EMTs were disinclined to allow me to hitch a second ambulance ride across the street, so I walked back to the clinic building and picked up where I left off.

Well now, an eventful beginning to one of my first clinic days as a surgical oncologist. It took most of the morning for heart rates of the staff (and me) to slow down to normal.

About nine o'clock the same evening my pager beeped and displayed a phone number I did not recognize. It was the patient's daughter. She reported that her father had undergone cardiac catheterization, which revealed several near-occluding plaques in three vessels of his heart. He had just been moved to the intensive care unit after urgent surgery to perform a three-vessel, coronary artery–bypass graft operation. The cardiothoracic surgeon had told her that her father was stable and he believed her father had not suffered heart damage.

Many patients have additional medical problems or disorders confounding their diagnosis and treatments for cancer. Frankly, it seems to me an increasing proportion of patients diagnosed with cancer have what we in medicine call co-morbidities. These conditions increase the complexity of cancer-treatment planning, and may increase the incidence or severity of treatment-related side effects and complications.

Diabetes is one example, but there are numerous medical co-morbidities oncology care providers must account for during the delivery of cancer therapeutics and surgery. High blood pressure affects one in three adults in this country. Hypertension increases the risk for heart disease, stroke, and kidney dysfunction. Approximately forty million Americans smoke cigarettes. This is a deadly addiction that causes numerous types of cancer, and is a major co-morbidity that increases the risk for pulmonary complications during cancer therapy, and impairs wound healing after surgery. This next statement is not intended as a bad pun, but as a grim warning: There is a growing problem with obesity in many countries in the world, with almost one-third of Americans classified as significantly to morbidly obese. Obesity is associated with increased risk for diabetes, high blood pressure, heart disease, liver inflammation leading to cirrhosis, and numerous types of cancer.

This is a reality of modern cancer care: patients have other medical problems or disorders. Even allergies to medications can become problematic. We may not be able to use a vital antibiotic to treat a difficult infection in a patient whose immune system has been compromised by chemotherapy treatments. Alleviation of pain or other symptoms may be limited by allergies to useful medications. Patients can develop allergic reactions to chemotherapy drugs, sometimes including a dreaded life-threatening reaction known as anaphylaxis. When allergic reactions to chemotherapy drugs develop, our ability to treat patients with the optimal combination of drugs intended to maximize the probability of long-term survival is necessarily hampered.

There are many clinical studies in the oncology literature indicating that medical co-morbidities have a negative prognostic impact on cancer patients. Some studies found cancer patients with one or more co-morbid conditions have a lower probability of long-term survival compared to patients with the same type of cancer and no co-morbidity. Additionally, some types of medical conditions reduce the safety of delivery of standard doses of chemotherapy or radiation therapy and may limit the options for surgical oncologists to perform a complete and appropriate oncological operation. Reports from the surgical literature worldwide have confirmed that postoperative complications and risk of death are significantly higher in patients with co-morbidities, and that these risks rise as the number and severity of medical co-morbidities increase.

When evaluating new patients with a diagnosis of cancer, we obtain information on all medical problems from childhood and adulthood, along with lists of any previous surgical operations, problems with anesthesia, unusual bruising or bleeding tendencies, and documentation of all medications and allergies. Treating cancer patients who have one or more concurrent medical conditions is commonplace; we focus on optimizing their cancer care while controlling and monitoring their other medical problems. The situation is what it is. When patients who develop cancer frequently have other medical problems, it is our job in oncology to develop treatment plans that account for the cancer and the additional conditions that exist or arise in our patients.

The gentleman in the well-worn overalls, Western shirt, and cowboy boots recovered well after open-heart surgery. I visited him several times in the heart institute while he recuperated from his operation. He was in the intensive care unit for two days and was discharged from the hospital nine days after the unplanned heart procedure. While he was in the hospital, I took his history and completed a physical examination. I also confessed to him that the single question and very brief examination of our first encounter were not typical, but his identified critical heart problem had become an immediate priority.

Fortunately, this man's rectal cancer was not obstructing his colon. He was eating normally and was not anemic, indicating an absence of prolonged or major bleeding from the tumor. The cancer was diagnosed by his physician after the patient had noticed some bright red blood mixed in with his bowel movements. Unfortunately, the tumor was very low in the rectum, overlying the sphincter muscles that allow us to control (hopefully) the passing of gas and bowel movements.

While recovering from his heart operation, my colleagues in medical and radiation oncology and I formulated a treatment plan for his rectal adenocarcinoma. Four weeks after his successful coronary artery–bypass graft operation, we began treatment with continuous intravenous infusion of a chemotherapy drug, 5-fluorouracil, or 5-FU, Monday through Friday, with radiation therapy to the area of the rectal cancer on the same days. He received this treatment five days a week for five and a half consecutive weeks, during which all bleeding from his rectal cancer ceased.

The cancer shrank after chemoradiation treatment but did not disappear. Four weeks after completing the intravenous 5-FU and external beam irradiation, the tumor was still readily palpable in a digital rectal examination and was visible when looking into the rectum with a proctoscope.

Cardiologists at the heart institute evaluated my patient and gave us the green light to proceed with an operation to remove his malignant rectal tumor. I performed an abdominoperineal resection, or APR, on this man six weeks after the final dose of chemotherapy and radiation and ten weeks after heart surgery. An APR involves removing a portion of the lower colon, the entire rectum including the sphincter muscles, and the tissue containing area lymph nodes. This operation requires creation of a permanent colostomy. For the rest of his life, this man, like all who undergo such a procedure, must wear a bag on his abdominal wall to collect stool exiting the colon.

This represents a really big, life-changing deal. Before the operation was performed, the patient, his daughter, a stoma nurse (an expert in managing the supplies, problems, and questions associated with a permanent or temporary exodus of bowel through the abdominal wall into a collecting bag), and I had a prolonged discussion about what a colostomy stoma would mean in terms of management and lifestyle changes.. We also had him speak with other patients living with a colostomy. Undeniably, he was not happy about the prospect of a colostomy, but he understood the oncological and anatomical constraints that warranted this curative-intent operation.

The surgical procedure was performed successfully, and no heart or other problems arose to disrupt his recovery. By the end of his inpatient stay, the gentleman and his daughter were comfortable with management of the stoma.

The preoperative chemoradiation therapy had produced significant killing of the patient's cancer. This major response to the treatment was good news and a positive indicator for the prognosis. The patient had stage III (lymph node–positive) rectal carcinoma, so he received six months of intravenous 5-FU and leucovorin. When I saw him for checkups during his chemotherapy treatment, he reported that the chemotherapy made him a little tired and his hands felt tender when he was driving a tractor on his ranch. Minor annoyances, he told me. Insufficient to slow him down, his daughter confided.

The man came to see me three times a year for a couple of years after his operation, and then every six months until we passed the five-year anniversary of completion of his cancer treatment. At that point we continued with annual visits. He told me unemotionally during several clinic visits that he disliked the colostomy. He had a wry approach about it, however, telling me a couple of years after the operation he had nicknamed the colostomy Bubba, because of its uncontrollable propensity to be loud and obnoxious at inopportune moments in public. He once told me, "Bubba has a lot more to say than I do." Bubba became particularly outspoken, effusive, and embarrassing when my patient drank two or three beers. The gentleman chose to quiet Bubba by limiting himself to a rare beer at a baseball game or an occasional scotch on the rocks during dinner.

Every time I saw my patient in the clinic, his outfit was similar. His standard attire was denim overalls, a Western shirt, well-worn cowboy boots, and a cowboy hat. I admit I assumed he was a proverbial good ol' boy from central Texas. He was a man of few words and expressed little emotion. He never put on airs and was deferential and impeccably polite to every member of the staff.

About seven years into our follow-up routine, his daughter invited me to an event in Fort Worth honoring her father. It fell on a weekend when I was available, so I accepted. I wondered what group was honoring this seemingly simple and soft-spoken man.

The event turned out to be a party for more than a thousand

people involved in the cattle business in Texas. My patient arrived wearing a tailored tuxedo, a black Stetson cowboy hat, and a pair of shiny Lucchese black lizard cowboy boots. From the look on my face, he could tell I was surprised and amused. He laughed and said, "I run a few head of cattle, Doctor." A few thousand head on several thousand acres, it turned out. This unassuming, undemanding, true gentleman owned one of the largest cattle operations in the state of Texas. Who would have known? We had a great time and raised money to support his two favorite charities, cancer research and a center for troubled young people in west Texas.

The gentleman rancher came to see me in the clinic for more than ten years. His daughter called me as he was approaching his eightieth birthday. The wear and tear of years riding in the saddle on working cow horses, bumping around in pickup trucks, and driving tractors and backhoes on his ranch had taken their toll. He wasn't getting around as well as he once did, so we agreed he would see his local physician. I received a Christmas card from this man every year for another five years until a note arrived from his daughter announcing he had passed away. His cancer never recurred. His daughter reported that while they'd had a tenuous and quarrelsome relationship at times, he had learned to coexist with Bubba.

I urge my patients with medical co-morbidities to do everything possible to manage their conditions well. Patients can take certain measures to help improve their outcomes after a diagnosis of and treatment for cancer: taking prescribed medications to control their high blood pressure, monitoring their diabetes closely to keep their blood-sugar levels in good control, exercising regularly and losing weight to avoid the problems related to obesity, and especially quitting smoking cigarettes if they are afflicted with that particular addiction. Coexistent medical conditions and unhealthy behaviors do more than increase the risk of complications and toxicities associated with cancer therapy; many medical disorders and personal choices directly produce conditions that cause cancer. Preventing cancer is always better than treating cancer.

Even Bubba wouldn't argue with that point.

20

It's Not Fair

"When you show deep empathy toward others, their defensive energy goes down, and positive energy replaces it. That's when you can get more creative in solving problems."

Stephen Covey

Empathy: The ability to understand and share the feelings of another

For a dozen years spanning the 1990s and early 2000s I had an avocation in addition to my career in surgical oncology, cancer research, and medical education. I coached my son's and daughter's soccer teams. My daughter was an avid player until she went to middle school, when she decided basketball, track and field, and music were more interesting. My son played soccer from the age of four through his college years. On his team, I had a core of the same players for a decade. A few came and went as parents were transferred to new jobs or as the players developed different interests, particularly once adolescence arrived. It happens. But by and large I had the same group of boys the entire time I coached.

When children are four or five years old, they play what I call piranha ball. The ball rolls to an area of the field and a group of eager children wearing uniforms in two different colors descend upon it, kicking madly. The ball eventually squirts out, the piranha follow, and the furious kicking resumes. Great fun with lots of laughter, and nobody cares about goals' being scored. The occasions when the ball ends up in the back of the net are usually random events amidst the chaos.

As my son grew older, it became clear that he was a good athlete and skillful player. He began competing on teams designated for more advanced players. Two evenings a week and every weekend in the fall and spring involved his soccer practice and games. His games took place throughout south Texas, and during his teenage years, included several trips annually to tournaments around the country. To assure I was up to date on the latest soccer coaching techniques, for two consecutive summers I accepted the extreme measure of living in a dormitory room for a week at the University of Oklahoma to obtain my United States Soccer Federation national coaching licenses.

The players who were on my team for many years came to know my idiosyncrasies. I had one notable pet peeve. When one of my new players committed a rough foul and was shown a yellow card, or conversely, when he believed he had been fouled but the referee failed to agree, he would come over to the sideline at halftime and complain, "It's not fair, Coach." The veteran players would moan, avert their eyes, and quietly creep away. Parents would clear their throats, grab their lawn chairs, and scatter. They knew what was coming: "The Lecture."

I would sternly ask the young man if he'd been granted a contract at birth stating life would be fair. Confused, wondering why he was deserted by his teammates, he would stammer out, "No." I would then affirm that life is indeed not fair and would provide examples of atrocities committed on innocent populations throughout history. I would go on to mention the fact that people, including children, without any good reason are diagnosed and die from cancer, and I'd state that there are children born with defects or who develop disorders that do not allow them to run and play on the soccer field. The Lecture would invariably end with, "Is any of that fair?"

Eyes downcast, kicking the grass with his soccer cleats, the player would quietly mumble an agreement that it was not fair. The chagrined and chastened player would wander off to join his teammates who would cheer him up, "Don't ever say that to Coach. He knows life is not fair, taking care of cancer patients."

The dust would settle, I'd give the player a pat on the back and a smile, and I would gather my team. We would have a rousing talk about tactics and some fun ideas for the second half of the game. It was a great time. My teams were always in terrific shape, and it kept me in good condition running and practicing with them. The kids played hard, clean, fair soccer, and I expected great sportsmanship from them. We won a lot more games than we lost. Those years coaching youth soccer allowed me to maintain a semblance of sanity when insanity swirled in the world around me.

I never displayed diplomas or professional awards on my office wall. Instead, every year I hung a framed poster of my team. Kids don't prefer to stand in straight lines, hands clasped behind their backs as in official team photographs. So instead, we posed wearing uniforms and sunglasses, while copping an attitude with a Harley-Davidson motorcycle or two in the background. Have some fun with it!

My football teams learned a lot of important life lessons and new vocabulary words (a daily ritual), and they realized soccer was a fun game. Win or lose, what counts is your character and how you conduct yourself through life. I learned from them, too. When my players graduated from high school, they and their parents showed up at my door one summer afternoon and presented me with a soccer ball signed by the entire team. They thanked me for teaching them perspective and an understanding of what really matters in life. For a rare moment, I was speechless. This is the only trophy or award of the dozens my soccer teams have won that I have ever displayed. Every time I look at that ball I am reminded what really matters.

Taking care of cancer patients is a daily reminder that life is not fair. Children are diagnosed with cancer. That's one the furthest things from fair I can imagine. Some patients diagnosed with malignant cancer have no identifiable risk factors. They don't have a genetic predisposition or family history of cancer, they exercise regularly, they do not smoke cigarettes, and they eat a healthy diet. Nonetheless, they develop some type of malignant disease. At some point during our conversations these patients understandably ask, "Why did this happen to me?"

I don't have an answer. Sure, medical genetics has advanced in its ability to perform somatic- and tumor-mutational analysis, which may detect key driver mutations leading to cancer. However, in most patients we don't know why DNA alterations arise. About eight years ago a woman in her early forties was referred to me with colorectal-cancer liver metastases. If you read the oncology textbooks, you learn colorectal cancer is diagnosed most commonly in the sixth and seventh decades of life. Thus, the current standard recommendation is to start screening with colonoscopy examinations at age fifty. This woman had no family history of colorectal cancer, or any other type of cancer for that matter. She developed rectal bleeding with bowel movements that persisted for more than a month, so she saw her primary-care physician. Subsequently, a gastroenterologist performed a colonoscopy and confirmed the presence of a circumferential colonic adenocarcinoma in the sigmoid colon, the last portion of the colon attaching to the rectum.

A complete evaluation including CT scans and blood tests revealed no other obvious site of cancer, so she underwent a routine sigmoid colectomy. Pathological evaluation of the specimen showed a cancer that had grown through the wall of the colon and had spread to three lymph nodes near the primary tumor. Colon cancer metastasizing to regional lymph nodes is classified as stage III. Several prospective, randomized clinical trials have indicated that six months of chemotherapy reduces a patient's risk of developing recurrent disease. While it lessens the risk however, cytotoxic systemic chemotherapy does not eliminate the chance that cancer will return. There are no guarantees. Instead, we play the odds to improve the likelihood of long-term overall and disease-free survival. After recuperating from her operation, this lady completed six months of intravenous chemotherapy, which caused significant side effects and made her lose time from work.

After recovering adequately from the toxic effects of chemotherapy, the patient resumed her normal life, and her medical oncologist saw her back in his office every three months. Nine months after finishing chemotherapy, a blood test indicated a possible recurrence of cancer, and a CT scan confirmed the presence of two tumor masses in the right lobe of her liver. At that point she was referred to me. At the same time, the patient's husband decided he could not deal with the stress of caring for a wife diagnosed with stage IV colorectal cancer, so he left her. That's not fair. I was presented with a patient bereft of comfort, frightened, and confused. After confirming with imaging studies that there was no evident metastatic disease at sites other than the right lobe of the patient's liver, I performed an operation that removed the tumor-bearing area.

One of the items I always discuss with patients before surgery is *recurrence of cancer*. This is a shadowy possibility we must consider and reveal. All patients go into a cancer operation hoping their tumor or tumors will be removed completely. Spoken or not, their wish is for a cure and the potential that their cancer will be nothing more than an unpleasant memory. But we surgeons know all too well that cancer may recur despite a sound, well-performed oncological operation and additional treatments with chemotherapy, radiation therapy, or other multidisciplinary approaches. Cancer is a consummate model of evolution. Malignant cells can adapt and mutate. Subpopulations of cancer cells with an advantageous phenotype can survive the hostile conditions instigated by toxic drugs, ionizing radiation, and other targeted therapies. These cells cannot only survive but thrive, grow, metastasize further, and wreak havoc in our patients.

After recovering from the operation, my patient and I discussed whether additional chemotherapy would be helpful. Unlike the results with node-positive stage III colorectal cancer, there is no definitive proof (meaning prospective, randomized large-scale clinical trials producing level 1 evidence) that additional chemotherapy after resection of stage IV colorectal-cancer metastases reduces the risk of recurrence. Nonetheless, this young woman was very concerned, and after weighing her options, she decided to undergo another six months of chemotherapy with a different regimen from the previous one.

This second combination of cytotoxic drugs hit her harder than the first round of chemotherapy she had received. She was hospitalized twice because of severe dehydration and infection related to immune suppression caused by the chemotherapy. She lost her hair, she missed significant periods of work, and her employer laid her off from her job. That's not fair. After completing her second six-month course of chemotherapy, we resumed the process of following her to watch for any recurrence of cancer. One year after completing chemotherapy, a CT scan revealed a new tumor in the left lobe of her liver. In this woman's case, subclinical nests of cancer cells were present in the liver when I performed her operation. We oncologists hope that chemotherapy will eradicate these microscopic areas of cancer, but the toxic drugs are not perfect and cancer can recur despite treatment. In fact, the drugs may actually lead to malignant cells that are more resistant to chemotherapy. That's not fair.

As my patient had already undergone two major abdominal operations and a year of chemotherapy, I discussed treatment options with her. I told her the single tumor could be surgically removed, and I believed this was her best choice. She considered it for about a week and then agreed to proceed. The third operation was difficult due to scar tissue throughout her belly cavity, but it was possible to perform a wedge resection of the single liver tumor. During the ultrasound examination, I found a second small tumor deep in the left lobe of her liver, which I destroyed with a radiofrequency needle. Once again, by the best tests and procedures available, she was rendered grossly disease-free. But because her cancer had recurred despite two different chemotherapy recipes, we agreed it was preferable to follow her closely and hold off on any chemotherapy or other treatments.

One year ago my patient passed the mythical five-year mark with no evidence of recurrent or metastatic colorectal cancer. She was elated. She had moved to a new city and had moved on with her life. Losing her job caused her to reevaluate her career options and she had found new, exciting, and rewarding employment opportunities. She enjoyed her work, co-workers, and friends and had time to spend with her family, including a new grandchild.

Life isn't fair. Six months ago I received a call from this sobbing patient. She informed me she had just been diagnosed with inflammatory breast cancer. She had noticed that her left breast seemed swollen and then rapidly it became hard and had areas of redness across the skin. She made an appointment with a medical oncologist in her new hometown and, upon examining her he immediately recognized the signs of an aggressive breast cancer. Radiographic studies and biopsies confirmed a second type of malignancy, unrelated to her previous colorectal cancer. The complete clinical staging evaluation revealed enlarged lymph nodes under her left arm, and a fine needle aspiration biopsy confirmed the presence of metastatic breast-cancer cells.

Inflammatory breast cancer is a particularly aggressive form of cancer, and her medical oncologist initiated a round of chemotherapy for this new problem. She recently passed, but did not celebrate, her fiftieth birthday. Understandably, she was not in a celebratory mood. None of this is fair. But it is the reality cancer patients face. The fear, the uncertainty, the painful and toxic treatments, the disruption of normal patterns of life, and the effects on family members and personal relationships are all too real.

I am not an expert on breast cancer, but I saw my patient back in my office a few weeks ago. It was a visit she requested more for reassurance than for recommendations about her current care. We talked for more than thirty minutes and at the end of the conversation, I confirmed I would continue to follow her closely and provide any treatment I could to help her. She shook her head and said sadly, "I don't understand why this is happening to me. It's not fair."

She did not get The Lecture. I gave her a hug and I agreed with her, saying, "You're right, it's not fair."

A few years ago a thirty-eight-year-old mother of four was referred to me to treat colorectal-cancer liver metastases. Four months previously she had presented with onset of severe abdominal pain and worsening constipation. Her physician ordered a colonoscopy that identified a nearly obstructing lower colonic tumor. An urgent operation was performed to remove the section of tumor-bearing colon along with the adjacent lymph nodes. The surgeon successfully connected the two ends of the colon together; happily, the patient did not require a colostomy. The surgeon palpated and then biopsied tumors near the surface of the liver, and the pathology evaluation confirmed a poorly differentiated, or aggressive-appearing, adenocarcinoma of the sigmoid colon with microscopic invasion by cancer cells into blood and lymphatic vessels. Several lymph nodes contained metastatic colon cancer, and the biopsied liver tumors proved to be metastatic colorectal cancer. She had just recovered from the colon operation and three months of intravenous chemotherapy when we met.

She seemed in excellent health, lean, robust-appearing, taking no medications, busy raising four small children, and she and her husband were avid cyclists. From a physical and medical point of view, she was a great candidate for surgery. Repeat imaging of her abdomen after six cycles of chemotherapy showed that of the five tumors in her right liver lobe, two had disappeared, and the remaining three metastases along with a solitary left-lobe tumor were greatly reduced in size. As usual, I discussed the indications, alternatives, risks, and potential outcomes associated with a major liver operation with the patient and her husband. After I finished she asked, "I know the cancer may come back, but it's not common is it? That wouldn't be fair." Ouch, the fairness thing again. We had a fifteen-minute discussion about the probabilities of cancer recurrence, and I told her the chemotherapy had produced significant shrinkage of her liver tumors, but I could not predict the future and could not assure her the cancer would not come back. She stated optimistically, "Well I've had all kinds of scans, CT, MRI, and PET, and the only thing that shows up is these tumors in the liver, so I think I will be fine." Combined wishful and hopeful thinking. I get it, but I reiterated several times that the cancer could return at any time despite aggressive surgical and medical treatment.

We proceeded and I completed an uneventful extended right hepatectomy eliminating all tumors in her liver except one small lesion remaining near the edge of the left liver lobe, which I removed with a wedge resection. All detectable malignant tumors were taken out with good, tumor-free surgical margins, and intra-operative ultrasound did not detect any additional liver cancers. The patient, her family, and I were all happy. A successful operation. While in the hospital she had the usual expected profound fatigue for the first few days of liver regeneration, but bounced back rapidly and was discharged on postoperative day five. I saw her in the office a week later, and she looked like she had just been out for a stroll. Her cheeks were pink and rosy, she had a big smile on her face, and she exuded hope and confidence. Her blood tests were normal, and I arranged for her to return to see both her medical oncologist and me six weeks later to discuss additional chemotherapy. The final pathology report on her liver showed only scar tissue where the two right liver tumors had vanished on her CT scans, and the remaining four tumors contained mostly scar tissue and inflammatory cells with a few isolated islands of cancer cells. Her medical oncologist was very pleased with the dramatic response to chemotherapy.

One week before her scheduled visit, however, she called me

and reported that during the previous forty-eight hours she had been developing increasingly severe pelvic pain. I instructed her to come to the emergency room immediately, and she and her husband were there within thirty minutes. She was clearly in severe discomfort. We gave her a dosage of intravenous pain medication and admitted her to the hospital. An MRI scan of her abdomen and pelvis was performed later that day.

When I met with her medical oncologist, we pulled up the images on the computer. We sat staring at the screen, astonished. The left lobe of her liver had regenerated beautifully, and the wedge defect where I had removed the left-sided tumor was readily evident. Also readily evident, however, were more than a dozen approximately one-centimeter-diameter, new liver metastases. The MRI scan of her pelvis revealed a previously undetected tumor invading the sacrum, eroding into the bone and pressing on the end of her spinal cord. Fast-growing early recurrences like these are not a frequent event, but when they happen it launches the entire medical team into a series of questions regarding what, if anything, we could have done differently to detect or prevent this situation. Often we have no discernible answers. It is a huge disappointment to patients, family, friends, and the treating physicians.

The medical oncologist and I entered her hospital room and had a long, emotionally painful conversation with the patient and her husband. We explained the findings and the need to engage our neurosurgical colleagues to first deal with the tumor in her sacrum, and then to initiate chemotherapy as quickly as possible. At one point, this woman looked up from her hospital bed at me and said, "You said cancer is not fair. You were right."

I wish I hadn't been.

One of our neurosurgical colleagues performed an operation the next day to remove the tumor invading the bone and compressing her spinal cord. While she had new surgical-incision pain to deal with, the severe pelvic pain had been treated effectively. After recovering from this surgery, she resumed chemotherapy.

She is still alive, but she has been on chemotherapy almost continuously for more than two years because her cancer stubbornly refuses to disappear and continues to pop up at new sites.

Cancer is not fair. Cancer does not care about fairness. But all of our patients deserve a fair shot at beating this dreaded disease. That's the promise. That's The Lecture I give them.

21

New York State of Mind

"Gentleness, self-sacrifice, and generosity are the exclusive possession of no one race or religion."

Mahatma Gandhi

Generosity: The quality of being kind and generous, sharing

Upon meeting new people and speaking with them for a while, it is not unusual for them to ask me, "Where are you from?" I know it may be impolite, but I answer their question with a question, "Why do you ask?" Invariably they respond, "You don't have an accent." I inform just-met folks that I was raised in New Mexico. This occasionally leads to a confused or startled expression depending on the individual's knowledge of geography. To erase uncertainty, I explain that New Mexico is actually one of the fifty states in the United States, not the country Mexico. Apparently my upbringing left me accentless but possibly, in the minds of some people, a foreign national.

All languages have regional slang, inflections, and dialects.

I have lived in Texas long enough to easily distinguish an east Texas drawl from a west Texas twang. Growing up, my impression and understanding of different American English accents came from television and movies. I was familiar with New Mexico Latino "Spanglish" and American Indian inflections, but prior to attending medical school I had not encountered people from the deep South or the Northeast, including places like Boston and New York.

Recognizing the location of an individual's upbringing by his or her accent is not a phenomenon unique to America. Scottish English is drastically different from American idiomatic English—and frequently incomprehensible to Americans. Even within a relatively small country like Scotland there are identifiable regional intonations. The whole of England is a fraction of the size of the great state of Texas, yet there are more than a dozen geographically based variations in pronunciation in England, from the Midlands, northeast, northwest, east Anglia, Yorkshire, southwest, and southeast. London may be considered separately with accents ranging from well-heeled aristocrats to proper BBC broadcasters to the cockney tones of the working class. Jolly good.

I learned from an unusual and unforgettable personal experience that languages other than English also have recognizable, and potentially inflammatory, regional differences. For more than twenty-five years I have been engaged in research studies in southern Italy. I spend at least one or two weeks a year in Naples at the G. Pascale Istituto Nazionale di Tumori examining the interaction between chronic hepatitis C virus infection and the development of hepatocellular cancer. I have learned to speak Italian well enough to wander the streets of an Italian city or town and get by with anything I need in the way of directions, information, or conversation.

Unintentionally but not surprisingly, I speak Italian using

Neapolitan slang and inflections. Several years ago, I was with two of my friends from Naples walking through the Palazzo di Caserta, the grandiose summer palace of the Bourbon kings of southern Italy and Sicily. It is opulent and remarkable in its architecture, artwork, and furnishings. Interestingly, the palace became a temporary Allied command center during World War II, after American forces occupied the region.

As my friends and I walked from room to room, we came upon a group of approximately thirty older Italians on a tour of the palace. These were people in their seventies and eighties, slowly shuffling along, some using canes or walkers, and listening to their tour guide. As we approached the group and started to pass them, an elderly Italian woman less than five feet tall spun around and poked me in the chest with her finger. "Sei Italiano?" (Are you Italian?) I replied, "No, io sono Americano" (No, I am an American). She spat on the floor at my feet and said in Italian, "You speak like a Neapolitan pig. Learn proper Italian!" I was incredulous and speechless. My two native Neapolitan friends were not. There ensued a chaotic and loud shouting match between the elderly tourists and my two physician colleagues from Naples. The tour group was from Bologna, and given the long history of enmity between various Italian city-states and regions, the memories run long and deep. The Bolognese were quite vociferous in their dislike of Neapolitans, who were not to be outdone and, despite being outnumbered, responded with a return barrage of obscene gestures and equally loud profanity. I shook my head and informed the entire crowd, in my best proper Italian, I was not involved in their centuries-old dispute. I bypassed the ongoing melee and proceeded onward through the palace. Mama mia!

In academic medical and surgical practices, our reputation for expertise and excellence in caring for patients with common or rare diseases is based on our reported outcomes and results in peer-reviewed journals. In the mid-1990s, I wrote a paper for a particular journal about surgical treatment of a rare type of cancer, called sarcomas, in the liver. Physicians and patients find papers like this when they are seeking treatment for an unusual malignant condition. My liver-sarcoma paper attracted the attention of a particularly interesting and entertaining couple from New York.

I returned from the clinic one afternoon, and my secretary handed me a note with the name and phone number of a man from New York City who had inquired about an appointment to see me. She said slyly, "Be prepared for an interesting conversation." Okay, a little mystery and anticipation.

I called the number and the patient's wife answered the phone. When I identified myself she immediately began yelling loudly, directly into the phone and thus, into my left ear, "Honey, Honey, it's Dr. Curley, get on the extension!" Within seconds, her husband, the potential patient, was on the line. For the next thirty seconds both of them, with thick, easily identified Brooklyn accents, a perfect verbal caricature of movies I had seen, spoke rapidly, loudly, and simultaneously, describing his medical problem. I couldn't make much sense of anything they said because they were both gradually increasing their voices to a shout to be heard over each other. Suddenly, the man screamed, "Dear, Dear, shut the @%&# up. I am talkin' to the doctuh!"

You could have scraped me off the floor with a spatula. I was done. I know it was not appropriate or professional, but I was laughing so hard I couldn't hide it. The couple on the other end of the line went quiet, and then the man started laughing, too. He apologized and admitted perhaps they were a little loud and excitable. A major understatement! His wife announced she would have more than a word for him once they were off the phone. Ignoring her remark, he promised they would take turns talking, which to their credit, they did for the next minute. Then, like flipping a switch, their conversation deteriorated to their baseline condition of two high volume exchanges going on at the same time.

After more verbal volley I finally learned that the man had an unusual malignancy called angiosarcoma of the liver. He had been told by several physicians in Queens and Manhattan that this was a poor-prognosis situation and that there was really no good therapy. After finally getting in a few words I asked if he could send his CT scans and biopsy results. The couple eagerly agreed, and I promised to call them back as soon as I reviewed the material.

These days CT or MRI scans come on a CD-ROM disk, but in the 1990s they were images printed on radiographic film. Back then, large packages with these sheets were routinely delivered to my office. This man's films and records arrived several days later. When I viewed the scans on a backlit radiographic film panel, I noted that he had a large hypervascular tumor involving the outside portion of the right lobe of his liver. I detected no evidence of any additional tumors in the liver or elsewhere. As promised, I called the patient and his wife, and told them I believed he was a candidate for surgical removal of this disease.

I can't describe adequately the shouts of happiness that ensued. After gathering themselves, the couple agreed to an appointment the following week. My New York patient and his wife appeared on schedule and they were everything I had hoped for. They were loud, boisterous, opinionated, and eager to give me a big hug and a kiss on the cheek. I am a tactile person; a hug from a patient or a family member always makes for a good day.

A surgical oncology fellow and I examined the patient and reviewed his options. We all agreed surgery was indicated. My patient and his wife flew back to New York to arrange for employees to manage their family-owned business in their absence.

When he returned to my hospital two weeks later, I removed the malignant tumor in his liver. CT and MRI scans are good, but still not as good as a surgeon's eyes and hands when he or she explores a patient's abdominal cavity. The only malignant disease evident on my patient's CT scans was the solitary liver lesion. However, during surgery I found two subcentimeter tumors in his upper abdomen attached to some fatty tissue. I removed both of these and he recovered from the operation without problems or complaints. The surgical unit staff loved him and his family. Every day when I went to check on him, and the nurses regaled me with the latest witnessed indecorous behaviors and sarcastic remarks between my patient and his family. They were, however, invariably gracious and thoughtful to the nurses.

Fuggedaboutit!

The pathology evaluation of the liver tumor and the two additional peritoneal lesions showed identical vascular sarcoma cells. I discussed the findings in detail with my patient and his wife, and I presented his case at our multidisciplinary sarcoma tumor board. All of his gross malignant disease had been removed, and there was no standard chemotherapy proven to reduce the risk of recurrence of sarcoma. Therefore, the board recommendation and decision was to follow him every three to four months with follow-up examinations and CT scans.

Bada bing, bada boom. The patient and his wife, sometimes accompanied by one or more of their grown children, would come for an appointment every three months. The entire clinic team and I always looked forward to their visits because we were guaranteed a vicarious moment of life in New York City with loud and unyielding opinions, arguments, sardonic comments, and a liberal infusion of four-letter words.

"You talkin' to me?"

Every time I saw this man, he would inquire if there was

anything he could do for me. He assured me anytime I came to New York, he would be available to provide transportation around the city, restaurant reservations, or any general assistance I might need. He had a genuine, generous, giving soul.

For almost three years my Brooklyn patient did well, working at his business full-time and enjoying his family and life. He and his wife thanked me effusively at every visit because they had been told by his physicians at home that it was unlikely he would survive more than one or two years. Therapeutic nihilism—our lives are finite, but all patients deserve our best shot at living as long as possible.

Unfortunately, cancer is cancer, and one month shy of my patient's three-year surgery anniversary, a single new liver tumor and another tumor in the belly cavity were detected on his CT scan. Once again, we discussed options including chemotherapy or surgical removal. He understood very well the side effects of chemotherapy, having had several family members treated for other malignant diseases, so he opted for a second operation. This was performed and both tumors were removed. Thankfully, the intraoperative ultrasound of his liver showed no additional tumors and I found no other sites of malignant disease in the peritoneal cavity.

Remarkably, this man's sarcoma never recurred. He went for another seven years with scans showing no evidence of new sarcoma lesions anywhere in his body. Sarcomas are known to have a high rate of local recurrence (that is, in the area of a prior surgical removal) and metastasis to the liver and lungs. Cytotoxic drugs to treat most sarcomas do not produce great results, so surgical removal of recurrent and metastatic sarcomas provides the best opportunity to control the disease and extend the patient's lifespan. In academic surgical oncology centers, we commonly recognize that sarcoma patients will educate a decade or more of our trainees about the management of these unusual cancers because many patients will undergo multiple operations to treat their disease.

Sadly, six months after one of his annual visits, my toast-of-Texas New Yorker's frightened wife called and told me something was wrong with his liver. She reported he had been feeling weak and tired for about a month, and was experiencing nightly fevers and profuse sweating. His physician in New York had ordered blood work, which showed markedly abnormal liver function. These same studies had been normal when I had seen my patient six months earlier. A CT scan performed in New York revealed odd-appearing nodules in his liver. The next day the couple was on a flight to Texas and I saw him in the clinic. I inspected his blood-test results and the CT images. The new liver abnormalities did not look anything like his previous sarcoma tumors, and there were enlarged lymph nodes around the great vessels in his abdomen. On physical examination, I discovered large, abnormal lymph nodes in his neck and armpit regions.

I arranged to remove a few of these palpable lymph nodes in the operating room two days later. After examining the nodes the pathologist diagnosed non-Hodgkin's lymphoma. It was a particularly aggressive subtype. I immediately referred this man to our lymphoma team, and they initiated treatment with aggressive chemotherapy. This worked well for six months and his enlarged lymph nodes and liver abnormalities disappeared. But he paid a heavy price for these results: his skin hung in loose folds from his face and body, he was gaunt and sallow, and his speech and movements were deliberate and pained. But he was defiant, "We fight on, Doctuh, we fight on!" His tenacity was inspiring.

Unlike his sarcoma, the respite from the lymphoma was short lived. Enlarged lymph nodes reappeared on CT scans, and he developed severe headaches only six months after completing therapy. Further testing confirmed his lymphoma had spread to his central nervous system. The next several months were painful for him, his family, and all of us treating him. He received intra-thecal chemotherapy, drugs administered directly into the cere-brospinal fluid flowing around the brain, spinal cord, and into the brain's ventricles. He had seizures. He was hospitalized numer-ous times because of severe side effects, immunosuppression, and infections related to the potent, toxic chemotherapy. He suffered headaches that were essentially untreatable by even the most pow-erful narcotic agents. On one of his admissions to our hospital, I visited him on the lymphoma floor. When I entered his room I found him literally hitting his head against the wall. I grabbed him and pulled him into a chair. Tears in his eyes he explained, "I am trying to knock myself out. I can't stand the pain."

Inconceivable. One of our tasks and goals as physicians is to provide our patients comfort and treatment for their symptoms. Everything the medical and pain-service physicians tried to alle-viate his maddening headaches was unsuccessful—unless they administered quantities so high he was essentially anesthetized. The problem with narcotic dosages that high is that people stop breathing; it is how someone dies from an opiate overdose. I have only respect for my colleagues who dedicate their professional careers to assist and treat patients struggling with difficult, occa-sionally intractable symptoms from chronic disease and associated therapies. They walk a fine line between controlling symptoms, and overdosage.

My New York kind of guy's lymphoma was progressing despite treatment, and predictably, and perhaps blessedly, a few weeks later he succumbed to his second malignant disease. Watching almost helplessly as he suffered was impossible and traumatic for his family and physicians. I develop close and lasting relationships with many of my patients, and this man and his family are among the most memorable. He was a large, jocular man who was effusive, demonstrative, profane, insightful, loving, and full of life. His glass was never half full but always overflowing. That overflow was a gift given to everyone he encountered, the overflow brought nothing but smiles, laughter, and joy.

We should all be so lucky.

22

Feeling Lucky?

"Have patience. All things are difficult before they become easy."

Saadi

Patience: The capacity to accept or tolerate delay, problems, or suffering without becoming annoyed or anxious

Most people are blindsided when they receive a cancer diagnosis. Folks are going about their business, living their usual lives, dealing with the joys, mundane tasks, and tribulations of modern life when "the big C" strikes. In some individuals, a new lump, bump, pain, cough, change in bowel habits, or other symptom develops unexpectedly and leads them to seek medical attention. Other people are asymptomatic and not diagnosed until they have a routine medical examination or after laboratory, radiographic, or diagnostic studies detect an abnormality. Examples of abnormalities in this latter group include a tumor seen on a chest X-ray or CT scan in a patient who doesn't smoke and has no cough or breathing difficulties, a suspicious-appearing spiculated, calcified lesion discovered on a routine mammogram in a woman who has no palpable breast tumor, or a colorectal cancer found on a screening colonoscopy in a patient who has no problems with constipation, change in bowel habits, rectal bleeding, or abdominal discomfort.

When I meet a new patient recently diagnosed with cancer for the first time, it is common for him or her to ask how or why they developed the malignant tumor. Not everyone asks. A person who has smoked two or three packs of cigarettes a day for forty years knows that smoking causes lung cancer. Patients with chronic hepatitis B or C understand that they are at risk of developing cirrhosis and liver cancer. And families or individuals with known mutations in specific genes are aware they have a higher risk of developing breast, ovarian, stomach, colorectal, or other hereditary cancers. For most cancer patients, however, the diagnosis is a nasty surprise. Seeing these shell-shocked patients, I have heard hundreds remark, "I can't believe my bad luck." It makes me think of a line from the song "Born under a Bad Sign" performed by the legendary bluesman Albert King: "If it wasn't for bad luck, you know I wouldn't have no luck at all."

One such unlucky individual was a man who was referred to me. Four years earlier, he had noticed some streaks of bright-red blood in his bowel movements. This had never occurred before so he went to his primary-care physician. A rectal exam showed no evidence of a palpable tumor, but the physician noted the patient had large hemorrhoids. He prescribed treatment for the hemorrhoids, but the patient's bleeding persisted for another several weeks. Recognizing this was unusual, his primary-care provider arranged for a colonoscopy. It revealed a circumferential, nonobstructing, bleeding tumor of the sigmoid colon. This gentleman was in his early thirties and had no other health problems. He was flabbergasted, as were his physicians. There was no family history of colorectal or other types of cancer, he had no history or endoscopic discovery of a predisposing inflammatory bowel condition or multiple colonic polyps, and he was much younger than most people who develop this cancer.

The patient was referred to a surgeon, who performed a sigmoid colectomy. The final pathology analysis of the colon and surrounding tissue revealed a tumor that had grown through the wall of the colon and spread to four of the sixteen lymph nodes that were removed. He was therefore categorized as a stage III colon-cancer patient. He received six months of standard chemotherapy, and was then followed every three months by his medical oncologist.

I entered the picture after this properly methodical and observant oncologist noted the patient's serum CEA level was elevated on the routine blood tests. A CT scan revealed four tumors in the right lobe of the patient's liver and one in the left lobe. The radiographic images showed no evidence of tumor at any other location in the body, so we discussed surgical treatment. Most patients are concerned at the prospect of any type of major surgical procedure, but this gentleman seemed particularly anxious. When I inquired about his concern, he reported he was having a run of "really bad luck." He was afraid he wouldn't reach the five-year cancer-free mark when he'd never have to worry about cancer again. That's an unrealistic view of the five-year mark, but I understand.

"If it wasn't for bad luck..." I had a long conversation with the patient and his wife and explained that the five-year disease-free survival target is not a promise of being cancer-free for life. He was despondent, but after further discussion, he and his wife agreed to proceed with surgical treatment of his colon-cancer liver metastases. I performed a right hepatectomy and radiofrequency ablation

of the solitary left-lobe liver metastasis. I always worry a little bit about patients who roll into a major operation with a negative attitude and a gloomy outlook. Those patients don't seem to recover as rapidly, and problems arise more frequently. This gentleman's operation went very well and he was recovering smoothly until he developed a fever on his fourth postoperative day. His fresh surgical incision was swollen, red, and angry appearing. The surgical fellow and I removed a few of his skin staples and pus poured forth. Fortunately, the sutures holding the muscle layers beneath the skin and fatty subcutaneous tissue were completely intact. The patient had a superficial wound infection. I explained to the man and his wife that we would need to clean and pack the area three times daily with sterile, saline-soaked gauze. The wound would heal slowly by what is called secondary intention. He gave me a look that combined exasperation and resignation, and then sighed, "More bad luck."

He recovered over the next few days and left the hospital. I saw him back in the office weekly and checked his wound, which healed well without any further difficulties or problems. His medical oncologist initiated a six-month course of a second combination of chemotherapy drugs. But the patient was only able to complete four months of treatment because of the severe side effects that developed. When I saw this man six months after his liver operation, he looked tired, haggard, and dejected. "Rode hard and put up wet," as my grandmother would say. Anxiety and depression are common problems in cancer patients, and should be addressed as part of their total care package. So I engaged my patient in a thirty-minute amateur-psychotherapy session that ended with me encouraging him to seek proper, professional mental-health counseling. He admitted he was not eating well or exercising regularly, he felt lethargic, and his sleep patterns were abnormal. These are common and expected symptoms of depression, but too frequently they're overlooked by physicians treating patients with chronic, debilitating, or life-threatening diseases.

"You know I wouldn't have no luck at all." Treatment of his depression and tincture of time improved the attitude and outlook of my still-under-forty-year-old, stage IV colorectal-cancer patient. Two years after his liver resection, at a routine office visit, I noticed immediately that his serum CEA level was again elevated. I quickly pulled up his CT images. His liver, belly cavity, and lymph nodes were normal. I switched over to the CT scan of his chest and observed two "new" lung metastases in the right lower lobe. I quietly uttered a couple of four-letter words at the images on the screen, collected myself, and entered his room.

He sat on the exam table, smiling, until he got a glimpse of my face. His smile turned into a frown, and I told him what I had seen on his lab studies and CT scan. He seemed to deflate before my eyes. Taking the proverbial bull by the horns, I told him he was otherwise in excellent health and would be a candidate for surgical removal of these tumors. After staring at the floor for about thirty seconds, he looked up and said resignedly, "Okay, what choice do I have?" I explained we had other options and alternatives available, but I believed surgical removal was best. He agreed, and a colleague in thoracic surgery saw my patient the same day. Two weeks later, my patient underwent a thoracotomy and surgical removal of the two lung metastases. No additional tumors were discovered during the operation. This time he recovered quickly and well, with no complications or problems.

When I saw him back in the office a month later he expressed mild surprise that the surgical procedure and hospitalization had gone so well. The patient's wife jumped in, "Stop whining! You're alive and for now you're cancer-free, let's get on with it!" All right then. The patient and I stared at one another, and we burst out laughing. I remember this conversation clearly; her remark was a verbal slap into thankfulness for my patient.

Two years after his lung operation, I saw him back in the office and it was clear he had lost weight. He remarked, "I decided to get serious about being healthier so I finally took your advice and I'm eating right and running every day." He mentioned that because he had lost about twenty-five pounds, he noticed a lump in his neck while shaving. I examined his neck; he had a palpable nodule in the right lobe of his thyroid gland.

Seriously? I explained we needed to evaluate this tumor. I ordered an ultrasound, which showed a 1.2-centimeter, solitary thyroid nodule. A fine needle aspiration biopsy confirmed a papillary thyroid cancer. When I saw him to discuss results, he looked at me bemusedly and said, "Okay, now what?" One of my endocrine surgery colleagues removed his thyroid gland the next week and my patient has been taking thyroid tablets every day for the last decade.

He doesn't talk about being cured of cancer anymore, but it has now been twelve years since my patient's lung operation for metastatic colon cancer. He received no additional chemotherapy, and no type of cancer has recurred since his thyroid was removed. He is appreciative and upbeat about being cancer-free for more than a decade now. During their visit with me last year his wife mentioned they have learned that patience and optimism can help to endure any tribulation they face. She is right. There is no serum blood test for a positive attitude, but in cancer care we have noticed that patients with an upbeat approach and a stable support system are able to bounce back from their treatments faster.

Not quite a decade ago, a fortysomething-year-old woman was referred to me with a diagnosis of a rectal adenocarcinoma and numerous liver metastases. When I entered the room to meet her, she immediately stood up, clasped my hands, and started crying.

"I am too young to have this cancer doctor. How could I have such bad luck?" I sat her down in a chair next to me and spent forty-five minutes speaking with her and her husband. After she composed herself, I was able to perform a physical examination. Her rectal cancer was very low and clearly involved the sphincter muscles of her rectum. Surgical treatment would require complete removal of the lower colon and rectum, and a permanent colostomy. The rectal cancer was causing her pain and bleeding with bowel movements but was not obstructing her intestinal tract. She had a fifteen-centimeter liver tumor involving the right lobe of the liver extending into the medial left lobe, and abutting the right and middle hepatic veins. There were more than ten additional small tumors in the right lobe of the liver and one located in the caudate lobe. This was bulky and extensive metastatic disease.

Strictly from a prognostic point of view, considering the probability of long-term survival, this was not a good situation. I was concerned about the size and volume of her liver tumors. Surgical treatment would become impossible if these tumors grew even a little bit while she was on chemotherapy or recovering from surgery for the primary rectal cancer. Other than having stage IV rectal cancer, this woman was remarkably healthy with no other medical problems or co-morbidities. I recommended, and subsequently performed, an aggressive surgical procedure the following week. I executed an extended right hepatectomy and caudate-lobe resection. This removed approximately 80 percent of her total liver volume. This large resection pushed her to the edge. She was in the hospital ten days after the operation and developed some transient jaundice. An operation to resect such a large volume of normal liver strains the functional and bio-chemical capacity of the liver. Some patients require infusions of fresh frozen plasma after an extensive liver resection because the small amount of remaining liver is not sufficient to produce clotting factors needed to avoid postoperative bleeding. In others, serum bilirubin levels rise temporarily and manifest as jaundice with the skin and eyes becoming yellow. Until the liver regenerates adequately, it is not able to process the bilirubin produced as a by-product of turnover and breakdown of red blood cells. Thankfully, while it was a struggle, this lady's liver regenerated and her blood work normalized after a few weeks.

Four weeks after her liver operation, while she was still recovering, we gave her a combination of low-dose intravenous chemotherapy and radiation therapy to treat the rectal adenocarcinoma. This approach required her to wear a chemotherapy pump Monday through Friday to receive a continuous infusion of 5-FU, along with daily radiation treatments Monday through Friday for almost six consecutive weeks. Her rectal discomfort and bleeding ceased midway through the course of chemoradiation treatments.

A month after she completed the chemoradiation treatments, I saw her back in the office and reviewed her new blood tests and CT scan results. Her liver had regenerated to an almost-normal volume, her liver function and serum CEA tests were normal, and the rectal cancer had completely disappeared on the scans and on *physical* examination. You know what I mean, right? Don't make me say it. All right then, on digital rectal examination. Sheesh!

Despite the apparent disappearance of her primary rectal cancer, there was a high probability that microscopic nests of cancer still remained in the wall of the rectum or adjacent lymph nodes. So the accepted, correct, standard-of-care next oncological step was to remove the lower colon and rectum and create a permanent colostomy, an abdominoperineal resection. I had a lengthy discussion with the patient and her husband. This lady, who had told me to "be as aggressive as possible" with her liver operation surprised me by saying, "I do not want a colostomy, and I do not want the rectal operation. I am feeling lucky."

I could not justify the patient feeling lucky as a bona fide reason to not pursue surgical and multidisciplinary treatments that were sound from an oncological point-of-view. But despite a prolonged and spirited discussion, the patient was steadfast in her refusal to undergo the operation. She did agree to six months of additional chemotherapy, which was subsequently administered. When I saw her back after she completed the additional chemotherapy, CT scans and blood work remained normal. I reiterated my belief that complete treatment should include surgical removal of the area that had borne the rectal cancer, and she repeated her refusal, telling me that she was certain that the rectal cancer was gone. In medicine, when treating patients, we provide our best recommendations, presumably based on sound clinical trials, evidence, and rigorous reviews of patient outcomes. We are human. And patients have free will and are not required to accept our treatment options. I recorded my recommendation and her decision to decline an operation, and we agreed that I would follow her closely.

This patient and her husband returned dutifully every three months for CT scans of her chest, abdomen, and pelvis, blood tests, and a physical examination. My colleagues in gastroenterology completed a sigmoidoscopy and endoscopic ultrasound of her rectal area every six months. There was no evidence of local recurrence of her rectal cancer. But eighteen months after completing chemotherapy, her CEA level rose slightly and a CT scan of her chest revealed two new lung nodules in her right lung. There was no evidence of tumor at any other site. She was, naturally, distraught, but she agreed with our multidisciplinary-conference recommendation to receive a second type of intravenous chemotherapy. She completed three months of the therapy and the two lung tumors shrank in size. After one of my thoracic surgical colleagues removed these two tumors, the patient completed another three months of chemotherapy and her follow-up resumed.

Initially, she did very well. For the next year blood tests, CEA levels, physical examinations, and CT scans revealed no evidence of recurrent or new metastatic disease. Unfortunately, a year after completing chemotherapy for the lung metastases, a CT scan showed two tumors in her left lung. There were no lesions in her liver, lymph nodes, or in the rectum. The word luck came up again. She stated, "I have not had good luck with chemotherapy, let's just take these out."

So be it. The same thoracic surgeon removed the two left lung tumors, which were confirmed by pathology analysis to be metastatic rectal cancer. She had already been treated with two complete standard courses of first- and second-line chemotherapy, so she declined any additional drugs or novel agents as part of a clinical trial. At her visit with me six months later, I happened to be standing in the clinic hallway speaking with one my colorectal-surgery colleagues. The patient and her husband were ushered from the waiting room into an examination room, and I introduced her to the doctor. He exclaimed, "Oh, you're the lady who won't allow us to remove her rectum! You are really pushing your luck." She glared at him icily and ended any further conversation or unsolicited opinions definitively, "I'll save my own ass, thank you."

No further comment needed. This patient's luck has not run out. She is almost a decade out from her initial diagnosis and has undergone and endured three major oncological operations and a year of chemotherapy. She has never required the recommended operation to remove her rectum and evidently the chemoradiation therapy completely eradicated her primary tumor. This is not unprecedented. Carefully conducted clinical trials with several types of cancer, including rectal adenocarcinoma, indicate complete pathological response and killing of all cancer at the primary site can be achieved with chemoradiation therapy in a subset of patients. However, we surgical oncologists have no way to distinguish preoperatively between patients who achieve a complete response following chemoradiation therapy from patients with subclinical areas of cancer still present. While it was not the standard of care, it is hard to argue with the outcome; my patient has survived almost a decade in spite of liver and lung metastases from her primary rectal cancer. And she has not had to live those ten years with a colostomy. Saved her ass, indeed!

Fate is fickle, fortune is uncertain, and luck changes. In surgical oncology and all cancer care, we strive always for excellence, but we like it if good luck is on our side. It goes along with the old saying "Better to be lucky than good, but best to be lucky *and* good!"

23

The Swimmer

"I know of no higher fortitude than stubbornness in the face of overwhelming odds."

Louis Nizer

Fortitude: *Courage in pain or adversity*

Growing up in the high Sonoran desert of New Mexico afforded my brother and me plenty of opportunities to run, play games and sports with friends, and bicycle across the mesas and arroyos around Albuquerque. Riding our banana-seat bikes on the sun-baked trails through creosote bush and piñon trees, struggling to pedal through the sandy bottoms of the usually dry arroyos, and pushing up into the foothills of the Sandia Mountains to then coast down at high speed was excellent aerobic exercise—particularly considering we were at an altitude of almost one mile. As an adult I continue to love running and cycling, and even competed for a couple of years in duathlon events that combined both activities.

I have never competed in a triathlon. There is a very simple reason: swimming is a not a forte of mine. New Mexico has an arid to semi-arid climate, depending on your location and proximity to the mountains. Until I was a teenager, the largest body of water I had ever seen was that great strip of mud known as the mighty Rio Grande River. Originating in Colorado, it courses north to south through New Mexico before becoming the natural border between Mexico and Texas as it flows into the Gulf of Mexico. I remember times when it flowed freely, particularly during springtime after a heavy winter of snow in the mountains, but for most of the year there was little water in the Rio Grande as it was diverted for the many irrigation needs of farmers along the river valley.

That is not to say I was not exposed to swimming as a child. My parents enrolled my brother and me in swimming lessons when we were very young, and we became adequate swimmers. Four or five times every summer we would be treated to a trip to the local community pool, called the A pool. The pool was constructed in the shape of a large, one hundred–yard long capital A. The flattened top of the A was the deep end and featured a spring board and a high dive platform. The end of one of the A legs was the "kiddie" pool, which we fastidiously avoided, and the opposite leg was the four-to-five-foot-deep swimming and playing area.

To my brother, my friends, and me, the most interesting feature was the center concrete island situated perfectly in the middle of the pool connecting the two legs of the A. This was an area to swim to, climb on, and cannonball or dive off in an attempt to splash our neighbors. This cavorting in the water was the extent of my aquatic skill and experience. The island was also a source of unending aggravation for the lifeguards. It was popular to play Capture the Island when two or more spontaneously assembled teams of kids would swim to the center of the pool and tussle to climb onto the island and claim ownership. This inevitably produced angry whistle-blowing from the lifeguards and shouts of, "Hey, you kids on the island, knock off the pushing and shoving!" Those clinging on to the side of the island would sullenly slide back into the water, while those already on top would cannonball into the pool as a wordless protest. There would be ten or fifteen minutes of relative peace as the groups of children would quietly reorganize, only to launch another assault for dominance of the island. The angry whistle-blowing and threats from lifeguards would recur numerous times a day. I don't know how they tolerated it; we were relentless nuisances.

In contrast to me, with my inefficient water-thrashing technique, I had a patient who was an excellent swimmer. He swam competitively for a top-ranked major Midwestern American university. He wasn't offered a scholarship, he walked on (or swam on, to be accurate) and showed enough talent and drive to earn a place on the team. After completing his university swimming career, he went on to earn graduate degrees and to work in the medical field. He was married with children and was enjoying his profession when he developed stage IV colorectal cancer.

This active and athletic gentleman was in his thirties when he was diagnosed. Another surprisingly young patient on the left side of the somewhat asymptotic age-distribution curve for time of detection. He had no family history of cancer, and during testing of his cancer and normal cells no genetic abnormalities were observed that would explain this early-age diagnosis. Nonetheless, he was faced with colon cancer and liver metastases. As is often the case with patients referred to me, he had already undergone surgical removal of his primary colorectal cancer and was receiving systemic intravenous chemotherapy. He had several metastatic tumors in his liver, including one that was unfortunately situated, abutting all three of the hepatic veins draining blood out of the liver.

I proceeded to remove part of the tumor-bearing right lobe of the liver, and performed radiofrequency ablation of the central tumor near the hepatic veins. This grossly treated all of the cancer we could detect. He recovered and received additional chemotherapy. But his cancer did not cooperate with our plans; it recurred. Within a year he had new liver metastases, including some at the edge of the radiofrequency-ablation zone, indicating that the tumor at this site had not been completely destroyed.

I performed a second liver operation. Once again, removing some tumors and destroying others with the heat generated during radiofrequency ablation. Based on the ultrasound used to examine his liver during the operation, all of the detectable cancer was removed or destroyed. I'll evoke a *Jaws* analogy, since swimming is part of this tale. Cancer is like the ocean, what's hidden beneath the surface can be dangerous. As already mentioned, the potentially deadly aspect of cancer is centered on the microscopic areas of malignant cells that remain and develop resistance to chemotherapy and other drug treatments.

The swimmer had these hidden clusters of cancer cells in his liver, and after lurking undetected for a few months, they grew to a size sufficient to be seen on CT scans. Bad words were muttered in the clinic. My colleagues and I responded with another barrage of chemotherapy, after which I performed a third liver operation. For the third time, I successfully removed or destroyed every tumor I could find in my patient's liver. He had no malignant lymph nodes or tumor nodules in his entire belly cavity. I should have been buoyant and hopeful, but I admit I was guarded and worried because three major liver operations and months of chemotherapy had not eradicated the swimmer's cancer.

Here was this former NCAA Division I athlete, skilled and self-motivated to compete at the collegiate level. He was intelligent and driven to complete graduate degrees and begin a career in a high-functioning environment, yet diagnosed at a relatively young age with stage IV colorectal cancer. Wouldn't it be nice if this story had a happy ending? Cancer causes many unanticipated, unplanned, unwanted, unhappy endings. This is a story about diligence, endurance, and persistence.

The fourth time metastatic colorectal cancer reared its ugly head in the swimmer was more complicated. He had recurrent liver tumors that were in difficult locations near blood vessels or bile ducts. Some could be removed, and others could have been treated cautiously with thermal ablation. However, more liver surgery was contraindicated because he had several small metastases in both of his lungs. We surgical oncologists have data that shows we improve a patient's chance of long-term survival when we are able to remove completely all primary and, for some cancers, all metastatic disease. My aquatic patient had too many lung tumors to remove, so he and I had several long conversations in which I explained why liver-directed surgery was not the optimal option. The swimmer was healthy and fit and received aggressive systemic chemotherapy instead. He searched and read extensively about novel approaches and different ways to treat cancer. He and I had numerous discussions about some of my laboratory research regarding the use of electromagnetic fields to fight cancer. My studies were all in the very basic stage of investigation, using cancer cells or animals with malignant tumors. Nonetheless, he was very interested and was motivated to find alternative methods to battle cancer.

The swimmer and his family initiated a swim-a-thon called Drown Out Cancer to raise money and awareness to fund cancer research. He did this of his own volition because he believed better approaches to treat cancer and reduce the side effects and toxicities of standard therapies were needed. My patient and other swimmers in his Great Plains community held a one-day swim event and raised thousands of dollars by swimming lap after lap to earn money people had pledged. The first year my patient swam to drown out cancer was about four years after his initial cancer diagnosis and well over a decade since his career as a competitive swimmer. When he informed me he had completed ten miles, I was speechless, an exceedingly rare state for me. I would have drowned myself after a few hundred yards had I attempted this feat.

The swimmer spent more time on rather than off chemotherapy after developing colorectal cancer. He received a variety of intravenous chemotherapy drugs, and realized the side effects were making it impossible for him to function in his medical career. Rather than despairing and decrying his bad fortune, he reinvented himself in an entirely different profession. He not only succeeded, he excelled, all while being treated with toxic chemotherapy agents. He had a clear set of priorities and made sure he spent time with family, friends, and others important to him. He was one of the most sanguine and focused individuals I have ever encountered.

Intravenous systemic chemotherapy was not working. The tumors continued to grow, particularly in his liver, where the majority of his cancer was located. So he entered an intensive experimental-treatment program. This required him to be hospitalized for three to four days every six weeks. A catheter was placed in the femoral artery in his groin and snaked by an interventional radiologist all the way up to the hepatic artery supplying blood to his liver. This allowed drugs to be delivered through the hepatic artery directly into the vessels going to the tumors. This increased the dosage of drugs delivered to the tumors while theoretically reducing the exposure of normal liver cells. The downside of this treatment approach was that for three or four days every six weeks the swimmer was confined to a hospital bed, unable to move to prevent the catheter from shifting or being displaced and causing bleeding or infusion of drug to organs other than the liver.

Imagine yourself prohibited from moving, sitting up, walking, or getting out of bed for *any* function for three or four consecutive days. The prospect would be maddening. For a former high-level athlete it was difficult, but he managed and endured the treatments. I would visit him in his hospital room, and we would talk about options, progress in my research, and other novel approaches on the horizon. I knew he was frustrated, but to me he always presented a stoic and calm manner.

Like most patients undergoing chemotherapy and other cancer treatments, this man suffered from significant fatigue and deconditioning. That did not stop him from swimming only weeks after receiving high-dose hepatic arterial infusion chemotherapy. I was mildly surprised when he called and told me he would be swimming in the annual Drown Out Cancer event. (He invited me to speak at the dinner that would take place after the pool activities. He knew my history as a kid from the desert and thankfully did not invite me to flail in the water.) He had not been training or exercising regularly because of his ongoing therapy, yet he swam ten and a half miles! He swam even farther than he had swum the first time he organized this fundraiser. Talk about an iron man! The night I spoke at the swim-a-thon event he was clearly exhausted, but he was exuberant. He had swum much farther than even he had predicted. I asked him how he had accomplished this feat. He thought a moment and replied, "This disease devastates too many lives. That thought kept pushing me to swim."

After several years of almost-continuous treatment with systemic or liver-directed chemotherapy infusions, the swimmer's

cancer became resistant to everything available and he succumbed. His brother sent me a note thanking me for my efforts
and for the time I had spent talking with the swimmer in the hospital room or on the phone. He also reported that the swimmer
had believed better treatments for cancer would be found, and he
asked me to keep working on new approaches to treat this dread-
ful disease.

I can't swim more than a few hundred yards before hauling
myself dripping and breathless out of the water. The swimmer,
in the middle of tough chemotherapy treatments, and with no
training, got into a pool and swam for miles. The spirit and endurance of cancer patients is an inspiration and testament to the willpower, resolve, and toughness of some people. And I do not forget
the family members, friends, and co-workers of patients afflicted
with cancer. They step up to support their loved ones, and endure
watching the rigorous challenges, painful surgical procedures,
side effects of medical and radiation therapies, fear, uncertainty,
and depression accompanying the shocking diagnosis and treatment of cancer. Everyone associated with a cancer patient is
drawn into the process of treatment, living in the shadow of the
disease, and, for too many, dying. They all are affected in some
way, and they must cope with a range of emotions and problems.

There are several new treatments reported in the last few
years making a big splash in cancer therapy. There are immu-
notherapies, drugs targeted to specific proteins or aberrant pathways in cancer cells, and personalized genetic testing to identify
abnormalities that can be treated with new or available agents.
Everybody—patients, family members, cancer clinicians, caregivers, and researchers—all hope for better methods to improve
the survival and quality of life for those afflicted with cancer.
We must continue to fund and investigate novel approaches to

understand, prevent, and treat malignant disease. To allow more patients to survive and thrive. The swimmer knew that clearly, and he and his family and friends did something about it. They swam to fund cancer research and "drown out cancer."

"Some days there won't be a song in your heart. Sing anyway."
—Emory Austin

Endure.

24

Things Get Complicated

"Life is a long lesson in humility."

J. M. Barrie

Humility: The quality of having a modest, rational view of one's importance

A surgical operation, whether major or minor, whether for cancer or for a benign condition, is not to be taken lightly. For an elective, scheduled operation, one human being is knowingly granting another human being, the surgeon, permission to cut him or her. Think about it for a moment. The implications are extraordinary. This represents an almost incomprehensibly high level of trust. It is incumbent on the surgeon to weigh and balance the risks, benefits, short- and long-term effects, alternative treatments, and possible problems associated with a planned surgical procedure. Patients entrust surgeons like me with their well-being and their lives, and ostensibly we all have the same goal: a good outcome.

Discussing a surgical procedure with a cancer patient is different from discussing an elective operation for a benign disorder.

Cancer patients are staring down the long-barreled gun of their own mortality, usually they've been confronted with this frightening reality unexpectedly. Cancer patients feel cornered and anxious, so they are willing to accept a recommendation for surgical treatment more readily than those deciding to address a nonurgent condition. Often cancer patients want the procedure done as quickly as possible. Caution and rational reasoning are replaced by fear and willingness to accept higher risks.

The most common question I am asked by patients and their family members is, "How many times have you done this operation?" Once I provide an answer resulting in nods of approval and general satisfaction, they ask few if any other questions. After I have ascertained that a patient is a candidate for a major abdominal operation, we choose a surgery date and schedule a preoperative visit.

The preoperative experience can be daunting. There are blood tests, electrocardiograms (EKGs), a brief physical examination, and consent forms to be signed—there are *always* several forms to sign during the preoperative visit. My approach during a preoperative examination is to review the patient's scans and blood tests with him or her, and all who are present in the room. Then I use charts, diagrams, and hand-drawn pictures of the liver or other intestinal organs to explain in common, easily understandable terms what steps I will take during the operation. I next go through a long list of potential complications. I often try to allay some of my patients' anxiety with an inane comment like, "Okay, now let's discuss the risks. As you know, I must go through the written list of possible complications on the consent form with you. I'm surprised it doesn't mention you could be struck by a meteor during the operation." I don't know if I relieve anxiety or cause more, but most people at least emit a nervous laugh or grin briefly. The number of potential complications is sufficiently unnerving and it amazes me that people don't exit the room visibly trembling. I explain the problems listed, and possibly some that are not included, are difficulties that may arise but have a low-to-moderate probability of occurrence—based on the patient's overall health status, presence of other medical disorders and medications that may increase the risks, previous surgical procedures causing scar tissue and alterations in anatomy, and the degree of difficulty of the proposed operation.

Once I have answered all questions and explained everything to everyone's satisfaction, the patient signs consent forms granting permission to proceed with the operation. At this point I have completed a surprisingly succinct discussion of the operation including the potential risks, outcomes, possible complications, and *imponderables*. This is a delicate euphemism linked to the other question I am occasionally asked, "What are my chances of dying, Doc?" Part of elective-surgical risk assessment and judgment includes choosing patients who have a low probability of a lethal event during or after the procedure. I inform my patients that the possibility of the ultimate bad outcome is exceedingly low, and assure them I will maintain a high level of vigilance and caution. I tell them, "I hope you will be stuck coming back to see me for a long time." This is the desired outcome, but not always the one achieved when cancer is a variable. After the visit with me, the patient is sent on for an evaluation by the anesthesia team with yet more discussions of risks and complications and, of course, another consent form to sign.

Surgery has frequently been compared to flying an airplane. Everyone wants to take off, proceed on the journey, and land safely at the planned destination, every time. When something goes awry, and someone is hurt or dies, it is always a serious, disturbing event, and all involved want to know what went wrong.

More than a decade ago, I performed a right hepatectomy in

a fifty-year-old man who had two colorectal-cancer liver metastases. His primary colon cancer had been removed two years
previously, and he had received no chemotherapy because the
primary cancer was small and had not spread to regional lymph
nodes, which were removed during the operation. During routine follow-up with his physician, however, two liver tumors were
discovered on his CT scan. He was an active gentleman who
walked daily. On weekends he rode his bicycle twenty to thirty
miles. He admitted he liked a glass of wine or beer with dinner
once or twice a week, but had never been a heavy drinker. He
had never smoked cigarettes. He told me he was ten to twelve
pounds heavier than he had been in college but he had recently
purchased a gym membership and was working out. He certainly
was not significantly overweight. Other than stage IV colorectal
cancer, his only medical problem was mild hypertension, which
was well controlled with a single medication. He had no symptoms, medical issues, pain, discomfort, or other disorders, and he
seemed like an ideal, low-risk candidate for surgical treatment followed by chemotherapy.

I performed the scheduled operation, and the procedure went
perfectly. The anesthesiologist and his team communicated with
me effectively during the process, the surgical fellow working
with me was skilled, and the entire operating-room team worked
harmoniously and seamlessly. We were humming along on all
cylinders, as my grandfather used to say. The intraoperative ultrasound showed no additional liver tumors so the tumor-bearing
right liver lobe was removed in less than two hours. He lost less
than a hundred milliliters of blood during the surgery, and all of
his vital signs were stable.

During operations, I always send word out to the patient's
family members and friends in the waiting room to give them
an update on how things are going. I know they are concerned

and fretting while I am working to remove the malignant disease from their loved one. For longer operations I might transmit two or three updates through the circulating nurse. But for a two-hour operation I provide a progress report approximately halfway through and then go out to the waiting area to deliver a full report in person after the procedure is completed and the patient is safely in the recovery room. In this fifty-year-old gentleman, I sent out a report about one hour into the operation to let his wife, children, and family members know all was going well and he was stable. As we completed the liver resection, I asked the circulating nurse to call out to the waiting room to let all assembled know things were "great" and that I would be out to speak with everybody in about ten minutes. The surgical fellow and I sewed up the muscle layers of the abdominal wall incision we had made to access the liver.

When we finished tying the sutures and started to close the skin incision, the anesthesiologist said, "What are you guys doing down there? His blood pressure just dropped." I looked up, over the sterile drape separating the surgical team from the anesthesiology team, and saw a blood pressure value of only sixty over thirty on the monitor display. The anesthesiologist asked, "Are you guys pressing on something or doing something?" I replied, "No, we just closed the abdomen, but something is clearly wrong." The fellow and I immediately cut the sutures holding the abdominal wall muscles together because I assumed a blood vessel or the liver edge was bleeding actively and causing his blood pressure to fall suddenly.

Nothing. The liver edge and the entire belly cavity was as dry as the Mojave desert on a summer morning. No active bleeding, no blood clots, no surgical issue to explain a rapid drop in the patient's blood pressure. At this point, the anesthesiologist called for assistance and said, "We have a big problem."

A major understatement. The patient's blood pressure went to zero on the screen and his heart rate, which had been 70 to 75 beats per minute, dropped within seconds from 40 to 20 to 0 beats per minute. No response was detectable from the EKG leads placed on the patient's chest. This is a condition called asystole; indicating no measurable electrical activity or function in the heart. I immediately began chest compressions as part of cardiopulmonary resuscitation (CPR). The anesthesiologist "called a code," initiating an inrush of nurses, support staff, and physicians into the operating room. The calm, measured, and pleasant environment from a few minutes earlier was replaced by barked orders for medications, harried placement of additional intravenous lines, and blood samples shuttled out of the room by sprinting orderlies to obtain laboratory results—STAT! I continued with chest compressions.

Fifteen minutes later, after alternating with other responders several times to apply CPR, I realized the patient's family must be wondering where I was. I was overdue for my appearance in the waiting room. I shouted to a nurse to call and let them know we were having a serious problem, another gross understatement, and I would be out as soon as possible.

Imagine how chilling that terse message must have been for the patient's family. It was miserable for the nurse to deliver it. I couldn't believe I was asking her to convey the information. The previous communication that everything was "great" should have provided a measure of relief and reassurance.

We continued our attempts to revive my patient for an additional forty-five minutes, following every accepted and appropriate cardiac life-support protocol, with different individuals rotating in to provide chest compressions as people became tired. I even went through the abdominal incision and opened the pericardium, the lining around the heart, and massaged the heart directly. The patient never regained any electrical activity of his heart and never had a return of any blood pressure.

After an hour, one of my anesthesia colleagues walked up behind me, touched me gently on the shoulder, and said, "I think it's time to stop. We've got no electrical activity." I was performing chest compressions at the time. I stopped and stepped back. I saw the flat line on the monitor from the EKG leads and the blood pressure of zero. Benumbed and disbelieving, I looked at the clock on the wall and said, "I am calling it. Official time of death is now."

The room went from loud, frenzied activity to silence and stillness. I walked past everyone who had come to help my patient, but nobody would look me in the eye. I took off my surgical gown, gloves, and mask and discarded them. I moved past the other operating rooms, gathered my white physician's coat hanging from a hook near my locker, and made the slow, long walk to the surgical waiting room. An operating-room nurse had called ahead of me to have the patient's family moved into a private consultation room. I walked in, closed the door, and said, "I am really sorry to tell you this, but he has died. Everything was going fine, but suddenly at the end of the operation his heart just stopped."

Before I got out the final words the patient's wife and daughters were sobbing loudly. All of the air seemed to leave the rapidly constricting, suddenly claustrophobic consultation room. I squatted down in front of the patient's wife and daughters like a baseball catcher and held each of their hands alternately, vainly attempting to offer solace. After a few minutes of weeping and whispered remarks of disbelief, they calmed enough to begin asking questions.

What happened? How did it happen? What went wrong? We thought everything was going fine, what changed? Why did this happen? I was peppered with a series of how, why, and what questions. I was shaken and stunned, too, but I maintained my composure and a professional demeanor. In retrospect, I think my voice was likely dull and monotonic. I gave an accurate and complete account of what had transpired and admitted I did not know or understand why his blood pressure had dropped precipitously at the end of the operation. Things had gone from smooth and stable to no heart activity in less than forty-five seconds.

For more than an hour I sat with them, sometimes quietly with no words spoken, sometimes responding to the next set of questions, which tended to be repetitive. But they had a right to all the time they needed from me. I eventually steered the conversation to a difficult topic when I asked their permission to perform an autopsy. I explained rotely that this was an opportunity for us to discern what had gone wrong and why an operation that had proceeded in a flawless, choreographed sequence, with no problems and minimal blood loss had ended disastrously, tragically. The family exchanged glances, and the patient's wife nodded and gave her assent. I handed each of them a copy of my business card with my office and cell number and asked them to call me at any time if they had questions or other concerns.

I was severely distressed by the experience; I had never had a patient die during an operation before. It has never happened since, but once was enough to burn a lasting impression on my mind. I didn't sleep that night. I lay awake for several hours mentally replaying the events time and time again trying to visualize anything that would explain the occurrence. I finally got out of bed and went to the kitchen table and reimagined every step, self-flagellating because I was not able to identify any unusual intraoperative variances or technical mistakes. I thought about every conversation I had had with the patient. What had I missed or failed to ask? I had gone through the standard "Review of Systems" questions about chest pain, heart disease, palpitations, breathing difficulties, reduction in exercise tolerance, and on and on, and all his replies had been negative. I specifically recalled a poignantly glib comment the patient had made during our first consultation visit: *"If it wasn't for this damned cancer, I'd be perfectly healthy."*

Late the next afternoon I received a call from the pathologist who performed the autopsy. The cause of the unexpected death had been identified. While the patient had no symptoms or signs of heart disease, including a normal preoperative EKG, the pathologist found an ulcerated atheromatous plaque at the origin of his left anterior descending coronary artery. This artery supplies blood to the beating muscle wall of the front side of the heart, including the left ventricle, which pumps blood through the aorta into all areas of the body. The vessel was severely narrowed and an acute clot had formed at the site causing complete blockage of this important artery. He had died of a major intraoperative myocardial infarction, a heart attack.

I didn't sleep that second night either. I ran the entire scenario in an endless repeating loop. During the day, I was distracted and withdrawn. Fortunately, I had no other operations scheduled for the next several days. I was able to push myself through a full day of the outpatient clinic and several research and administrative meetings, trying to maintain a veneer of normalcy. I reviewed the patient's medical record several times, wondering what I could or should have done differently. He had completely asymptomatic but critically dangerous coronary-artery disease. Were there signs I missed or should have detected?

I called his wife and family and explained the autopsy findings. I reported that I was surprised because he had had no symptoms or clinically evident findings of an impending heart attack. Acute blockage of the left anterior descending coronary artery is a common cause of sudden death; cardiologists call it the widow maker.

The patient's wife was incredibly gracious and thanked me for the information and for my attempt to help her husband by performing an operation to rid him of the cancer.

The next week my patient's case was presented at our weekly Morbidity and Mortality, also known as M&M, conference, in which we discuss any complication or death that occurred during or after an operation. Customarily, a surgical resident or fellow involved in the procedure presents the patient's information, describes the complication, and reviews surgical literature on the specific condition and operation, including any reported earlier complications and their subsequent management. The M&M conference is a surgical tradition. These days the meetings are much calmer and kinder than the ones I attended as a surgery resident more than twenty-five years ago, but M&M is and should be an open and honest disclosure to our surgical peers, trainees, and students of any complication or death that occurred during or after an operation. After the primary surgeon and the resident or fellow lay out the facts and findings, we await an unflinchingly direct review from our colleagues with comments, suggestions, and discernment of what could and should have been done differently. In order to understand the genesis of a complication and to avoid a recurrence of the situation in the future, we often categorize problems as: technical mistakes, errors in judgment, misdiagnosis, or delayed diagnosis. It is an important educational episode with an opportunity for all present to learn from earnest and forthright discussions on improving our patient care and surgical outcomes. The fellow involved in the operation with me gave a succinct but thorough presentation, including projected slides of the patient's CT scans showing his liver tumors, his normal preoperative blood tests, and his normal preoperative EKG. The fellow also provided a verbal description of the operation and terminal events.

After the fellow finished speaking the room was silent. There were no pearls of wisdom to be gained from my peers or colleagues. One of the senior surgeons sitting in the middle of the room turned to me, sitting sullenly in the back row of the small auditorium, and stated plainly, "I know this is tormenting you, but things sometimes happen you can't predict or alter. This man had no symptoms warning you about critical coronary-artery disease, and there is no obvious reason why it occluded at the end of your operation."

M&M conference can be somewhat humiliating and humbling, or it can be cathartic. This conference was neither for me. My senior colleague's comments were sympathetic, but I was not comforted. None of us could detect a technical error, an equipment malfunction, a preoperative-assessment omission, or a mistake in judgment. It was what it was. Reports in surgical scientific literature regarding techniques and outcomes for a variety of procedures inevitably include a list or table with rates of complications and mortality. That is why, for some surgeons, complications and deaths are reduced to a statistical event, an austere and unfeeling probability, and they sometimes adopt a perspective that may be too dispassionate. This is not, and should not be an accepted reality because a surgical complication affects the patient, the family and caregivers, the surgeon, and the entire surgical team. Ultimately, after several days of excessive and unhealthy self-torment, I realized I had to grieve, accept, exercise (run) to blow off some angst, and allow myself to heal over time.

For high-acuity (meaning difficult, technically demanding, unusual, or dangerous) operations, reports in surgical journals repeatedly indicate that the results are better when the procedure is undertaken by surgeons who perform the operation routinely. The results are better regarding complication, mortality, and survival rates of patients. An additional important factor in the improved-outcome equation is that the operations are performed in hospitals that provide care for large numbers of patients undergoing the operation. This is certainly true for many advanced surgical oncology procedures. But no surgeon and no medical center is perfect. Every time I meet with a patient and his or her family and review the list of potential complications and problems that may arise after an operation, I quietly hope and pray the patient will recover well and uneventfully. I have learned in harsh lessons to remain vigilant because problems can arise to blindside us just when we think all is well.

One of the complications we fear after surgery is deep venous thrombosis, or DVT, which is blood clots forming in veins. Cancer patients may have a higher risk of developing this complication than other surgery patients do. In a worst-case scenario, the blood clot can break free from a vein in the leg or pelvis and travel through the heart to the pulmonary arteries and cause a blockage called a pulmonary embolus, or PE. This can trigger shortness of breath, low oxygen levels in the blood, or sudden death. A few years ago, I operated on a sixtysomething-year-old businessman from an Eastern coastal state. He had a solitary right-lobe intrahepatic cholangiocarcinoma. He was an avid sportsman who enjoyed hiking, camping, and fishing. He ran two to three miles daily. He was in excellent physical condition and had no other medical problems when I performed a routine right-liver resection on him. Pre- and postoperatively we treated him prophylactically with subcutaneous injection of an anticoagulant medication to reduce the risk of blood clots. The operation went well with a blood loss less than 150 milliliters. He was up walking laps around the nursing unit the night of the surgery. On postoperative day four he was discharged from the hospital. When I saw him a week later in my clinic he expressed his sincere appreciation, he reported he was feeling well and was ready to return home. We set an appointment for him to see me six weeks later with blood tests and a CT scan to assess his liver regeneration and overall progress before beginning chemotherapy.

Two weeks prior to his scheduled visit, his wife left a message at my office. I saw the note on my desk when I returned from the clinic. I called her and cheerfully said, "Hi, how's everything going?" My ebullience immediately disappeared when she said, "I'm sorry to tell you, but I have bad news." She told me her husband had gone that morning to sit in a lawn chair overlooking a lake on the back of their property in the foothills of the mountains. This was his long-standing ritual and he would relax with his Labrador retriever and a cup of coffee enjoying the view as the sun and mist rose over the water. When he failed to come in for his routine shave and shower before going to work, she walked out to check on him. The dog was sitting beside him, his chin resting on my patient's arm. She spoke to her husband as she walked up behind him, and when he didn't reply, she noticed he was slumped sideways in his chair. She came around in front of him, and realized he was dead.

I was staggered, but then asked what I could do for her. I discerned from her voice that she was in the peculiar disbelief phase that often follows an unanticipated event. She told me that all she wanted was an answer to what had happened. She informed me she had agreed to an autopsy because she didn't understand why he had died suddenly when he was recovering well and had returned to work and normal activities. A few days later, the referring medical oncologist called to inform me that my patient had suffered a major pulmonary embolus.

I was dumbfounded—but also angry. The entire medical team and I had followed all of the current and recommended guidelines and protocols. We treated him with anticoagulation medicine before and after the operation, and he was still on this medication at the time he developed the blood clot that traveled to his lungs and killed him. How the hell had this happened despite our adhering to the correct DVT-prevention treatment protocols? Maddening! This patient's untimely death reminded me of a harsh reality of surgical practice. Numerous publications and studies note that the incidence of DVT and PE after major surgical operations is *reduced* by proper use of anticoagulation medications, but it's not eliminated. We are like Las Vegas bookmakers: we calculate and assess odds and intervene in an attempt to lower risks and influence fate, but there are no guarantees. Complications may arise despite thorough assessment, a well-performed operation, and adherence to all preventative measures.

Patients are willing to accept significant risks to undergo an operation to remove their malignant disease. Nonetheless, when those potential risks materialize as problems affecting the length of hospitalization, quality of life, or even survival, it is a disturbing, painful, and frustrating occurrence for all involved. Surgeons continue to search for ways to reduce risk profiles, but complications are the ghosts in the machine, lurking and appearing to disrupt a patient's course and treatment plans.

I obsess and worry about any patient I treat who develops a complication. When I was a surgical resident, the vice chairman of surgery, a man I deeply respected and who was very important in my surgical training, pulled me aside, and said, "You need to be careful. You get too involved, and you care too much." While I understood the remark, I admit I stared at him with some incredulity and responded, "I don't know how else to take care of our patients. If I stop feeling, it will be time for me to stop doing this."

I'm not planning to stop any time soon.

25

The Golfer

"Everyone should be respected as an individual, but no one idolized."

Albert Einstein

Respect: A feeling of deep admiration for someone or something elicited by the person's abilities, qualities, or achievements

Golf is a peculiar game. I occasionally watch the standup-comedy routine by the late comedian Robin Williams describing, with a heavy Scottish brogue, of course, the origins of the game in Scotland. Not only is it funny, but it rings true. His explanation that each swing of the club is called a stroke because frequent frustration and errant shots make the average golfer feel like he or she is having an actual stroke is an inspired etymology. I always find it odd but entertaining to watch grown men and women thoughtfully choosing a long metal or graphite stick attached to a variably angled piece of metal to hack away, some much more gracefully than others, at a small white ball, hoping to control its destination.

Even the most skilled golfers, those who earn a living playing the game, hit a fair number of shots that end up in all the wrong places. Like the beach, also known as a sand trap; or the rough, devilishly long grass that seemingly engulfs and grasps the ball. Or the woods, an interesting and potentially dangerous opportunity for self-injury caroming the ball off trees like a ball in a pinball machine; or the water, where the ball splashes down like the capsule at the end of an Apollo space flight.

I am not a good golfer. I play six or seven times yearly. It is unusual for me to find four or five hours of time on a pleasant day to go out and chase a little white ball through the high grass, trees, and back yards of the people unfortunate enough to live on a course where I happen to play. However, I am guaranteed four rounds of golf annually. Every spring I partake in a hallowed tradition. I go to Las Vegas with three friends and fellow surgeons from Chicago suffering from severe cabin fever related to the long cold winter in their Lake Michigan–side city. The sum total of our sins in Sin City is to play four consecutive days of bad golf, eat more red meat in four days than we eat in the four months before the trip, and talk so much trash and laugh so hard that we return to work the next week hoarse.

Bad golf for us means losing a dozen or so golf balls in the desert or rocky arroyos running alongside a perfectly cut fairway. If one of us breaks 100 it is a cause for major celebration, and a reason to require the offender who earned a respectable double digit score (without mulligans) to buy drinks for all at the nineteenth hole. All four of us were athletes in our younger years but never found the time to become skillful at the game. I emphasize I cannot bring myself to call golf a sport. I am hard pressed to designate an activity a sport when there is a person who drives around the course to provide snacks and beverages, both alcoholic and otherwise, while playing the game. And riding from shot to shot in a golf cart, this is exercise?

A few years ago my friends and I played a new course in Las Vegas that was much too fancy and difficult for our group. We were required to take a caddy with us, which was not something we had ever previously done. On the first hole he politely explained where we should place our tee shots to be well positioned for a second shot. Our group glanced at one another and each proceeded to tee off and strike the ball. At the conclusion of four opening shots that landed nowhere close to the caddy's recommended destination, we looked at him and said, "Your job today is to help us find the balls after we hit them into random and unpredictable locations." He nodded and maintaining a calm, professional demeanor stated, "I get it. Game on!" Good sport! Plus, he did need to think about his tip at the end of the day, so laughing at us could have had an undesirable consequence.

Occasionally, I have a patient semi-jokingly ask if I plan to play a round of golf after I complete an operation. There are still plenty of people who believe doctors spend lots of time on the golf course. Perhaps there are some who do, but I am not one of them. I explain to patients I am only invited onto nice golf courses if they have a need to aerate their usually well-groomed lawns. I also admit I have a tendency to annoy the serious golfers because I spend a great deal of time boisterously laughing or faux-contemptibly commenting about my own wildly errant shots. It is not uncommon for my Chicago-based surgical friends or me to note sarcastically after one of us strikes the ball, "Hey, nice shot; you're in the fairway." The problem is, frequently it's the fairway for the next hole. And out of bounds? We created an entirely new definition for hitting balls out of bounds. We need a bullhorn to shout, "Fore!"

Some years ago, a new patient asked me if I played golf. I explained I was an occasional golfer and not at all proficient at the game. I remember the conversation vividly.

PATIENT: What's your handicap?
ME: The clubs, the balls, and the golf courses.
PATIENT (laughing): I understand.

And I knew he did.

I asked him if he played, and to my surprise he replied, "Yes, I'm a professional golfer." He went on to tell me he was the Professional Golf Association (PGA) player and instructor at a course in a well-known East Coast golf destination. I was impressed, but told him we would talk about his cancer-related issues first and perhaps sometime later he could offer advice on my golf swing. This was an agreeable arrangement and he appreciated my prioritization of problems.

I met this gentlemen and his wife three years after he was diagnosed, in his early thirties, with a rare situation, a carcinoid tumor of his bile duct. This tumor had been removed at another institution but as carcinoid tumors frequently do, the cancer had putatively reappeared in his liver. His treatment had involved removal of the bile duct and reattachment of his liver bile ducts to a loop of bowel and, subsequently, six weeks of radiation therapy. Ionizing-radiation treatments to the base of the liver are not without risks. Proving the saying "No good deed goes unpunished," the radiation therapy to prevent recurrence of his bile duct carcinoid tumor caused a significant problem: he developed bleeding and pain from a duodenal ulcer which required treatment. Fortunately, the ulcer resolved with intensive antacid therapy and tincture of time.

When we met, the golfer brought CT images suggesting the presence of small, new tumors in his liver. The scans showed a couple of really small nodules not definitive for recurrent cancer, and he had no evidence of carcinoid syndrome. After obtaining new imaging studies, we decided to follow him closely and not intervene with any therapies until he showed signs of obvious tumor growth or developed symptoms.

Over the next several years not much happened. We continued to detect a couple of small spots on his liver with CT scans, but the spots didn't grow or change in appearance. Nothing new developed in his liver or elsewhere. He was still playing golf and functioning normally. His blood and urine tests showed no endocrine symptoms or biochemical evidence of hormone overproduction. Things were stable, and he felt well. So we watched.

Patients who have cancer can have other medical problems arise. About eight or nine years into our relationship the golfer developed severe jaw pain. He saw a physician who diagnosed him with temporomandibular joint (TMJ, the hinge joint where the lower jaw connects to the skull) dysfunction. The pain persisted and worsened so his doctor ordered a CT scan of his head and neck region. At this point I received a call from the golfer's wife to report he had been admitted with a dissection of his right carotid artery. This means a small tear had formed in the innermost lining of the large artery (the one with a pulse that can be felt on either side of the neck). When this happens, blood is able to enter the space between the inner and outer layers of the vessel, causing narrowing or complete occlusion, which can cause a major stroke. This would be disastrous for anyone, let alone a fortysomething, active professional golfer.

Thankfully, he had no neurologic consequences beyond local pain related to the arterial dissection; the jaw pain was caused by reduced blood flow to the muscles and tissues of the jaw. The arterial problem was addressed and the symptoms resolved. The golfer's wife asked if carotid-arterial dissection was associated with carcinoid tumors. I explained I had never encountered such a problem in a carcinoid patient but promised to get back to her after doing some research.

My research showed no propensity toward carotid, or other, arterial dissections in patients with carcinoid tumors. And the golfer did not have high blood pressure or other risk factors for arterial dissection. When I next saw him in the office, I happily reported there was no change in the small, asymptomatic liver tumors on his CT scans. Sardonically, I added he just had to be different and develop an arterial dissection to cause increased bother and worry. With his customary wry smile he retorted that the "unusual was usual" for him.

I have only a single patient who is a professional golfer, but I have met one other somewhat recognizable golf pro. Someone you may have heard of: Arnold Palmer. We met seven or eight years ago because he is a friend of a great guy I was collaborating with, Jim Rutkowski Sr., from Erie, Pennsylvania. Jim knew I was giving a medical lecture in Florida so he arranged for me to meet Mr. Palmer. I had dinner with Mr. and Mrs. Palmer at his golf course in Orlando, Bay Hill. He told great stories and we had a marvelous time.

Later the same year he came to Houston as host of a Senior PGA Tour event. Thoughtfully, he called and invited me to lunch at the course during the tournament. We dined and then walked out to check on the proceedings. We didn't get far because every few steps a fan would deferentially ask for an autograph or photo with Mr. Palmer. It took us thirty minutes to walk fifty yards. He was kind, patient, and turned nobody away. He smiled for pictures and signed balls, caps, shirts, and programs along the way until we finally arrived to watch the shots land on (or near) the eighteenth green. I found him a noble, considerate, and wonderful man, and I greatly enjoyed our conversations.

A few years ago he asked me to visit him again in Orlando two weeks before his annual (Bay Hill) Invitational PGA Tournament. I took my father-in-law, one of the aforementioned serious golfers, and he and I played two rounds. On the practice tee the second day, Mr. Palmer quietly ambled up behind me and watched a few shots. He asked, "Can I give you some advice, Doctor?" *Are you kidding? Free golf advice from Arnold Palmer!* I readily accepted his offer, and with a solemn face he said, "Don't give up your day job." He slowly walked away, laughing. Thank you, Mr. Palmer. By the way, the rough at Bay Hill was so long I lost four golf balls in two days on shots that simply rolled from the fairway into the long grass. It was as if the balls had crossed the gravitational field of tiny black holes that had sucked them into the weeds, never to be seen again. How do those professionals hit out of the stuff?

About five years ago, my professional golf patient had another strange medical event. He developed a large abscess in the right lobe of his liver. He had fever, chills, and upper-abdominal pain. CT imaging revealed an area of infection in his liver. It was not clear if the area represented an infected tumor or some other cause. A drain tube was placed through the skin into the infected fluid in his liver, and he was placed on high doses of intravenous antibiotics.

I reviewed the CT images with a radiology colleague, who was worried that the infection might have arisen in one of the small tumors and progressed into a large, dangerous abscess. The golfer was still having symptoms, and I wanted to control the infection because of the direct connection between his bile duct and a loop of his intestine. I discussed and considered options with the golfer and his wife. Concerned about infected tumor tissue, which may not heal or resist infection like normal tissue, we came to an agreement, and I removed the right lobe of his liver. The intraoperative ultrasound revealed he had evidence of ongoing inflammation and what appeared to be small tumor nodules around and near the liver-abscess cavity. However, he persisted with his medically unusual propensities and the final pathology showed only an abscess of the liver with no tumor in any spot in the liver, carcinoid or otherwise. He recovered well, and thankfully has had no recurrence of any odd infections in the liver, nor at any other site. His wife and I are waiting cautiously. There's no telling what he'll do next.

Carcinoid and some other neuroendocrine cancers can be odd actors and patients can survive with the disease for many years. It's been almost twenty years since the golfer was diagnosed with carcinoid cancer. He moved a few years ago from the seaside golf resort to another beautiful location in the Appalachian Mountains. He serves as the full-time PGA professional at his new job and golf course. About three years ago he developed some of the classic symptoms of carcinoid syndrome. He started flushing as many as fifteen times a day and was having loose bowel movements. For the first time, his blood-test levels measuring carcinoid-tumor-related hormone production were very elevated. Despite the symptoms, we saw no obvious tumors in his liver or elsewhere, but microscopic deposits of carcinoid-cancer cells within the liver can release the excess hormone. Despite the absence of detectable tumor nodules, the noxious carcinoid symptoms were negatively impacting his life, and I started him on a once-monthly injection to block the effect of the excess hormone release. He has thanked me for controlling the symptoms, but he also informed me I've become a real pain in his butt. The agent is injected in a relatively large volume with a long, hefty needle directly into the gluteus maximus muscle. Left cheek one month, right cheek the next, repeat indefinitely. You are welcome.

The golfer is a thoroughly pleasant and persistently patient individual. I have benefited from the lesson his patience has taught me. He is unflappable and implacable—characteristics I must remind myself daily to seek and achieve. After caring for him for many years, his wife informed me that he had independently initiated an annual marathon-golf event to raise awareness of cancer and money for research. This requires him to play hole after hole of golf for twelve to fourteen consecutive daylight hours. He has been marathon-golfing and attracting pledges per hole for about a decade now. He has played between 99 and 127 holes in a single day. Yet he golfs on, living with his cancer, and has gone the extra distance to help fund research. Fore to cancer!

The golfer accepts and lives with his carcinoid disease. Interestingly, when he comes to see me twice a year we still are not able to detect any carcinoid tumors on CT or MR images of his chest, abdomen, or pelvis. We know the cells are there, however, because his serum hormone levels are still elevated and he develops severe symptoms if he doesn't receive his monthly pain-in-the-butt injection. The treatment doesn't stop him from maintaining his coy smirk and enjoying his daily life. And, as he told me, he gets to earn a living playing a game, so what does he have to complain about? I can't argue with that.

A few years ago, I happened to see the golfer a few weeks before my annual Las Vegas golf junket with the boys from Chicago. I told him I should probably come to him for lessons, and courteously he said, "Well, show me your swing." I addressed an imaginary golf ball on the examination room floor, executed my back swing and down swing through the ball, and finished with a follow-through flourish. I looked at him expectantly. He nodded thoughtfully, shook his head and said, "You know, some things just can't be fixed." And then he laughed heartily. Payback, Baby, for the pain I caused him!

I'm now two for two on acerbic remarks from golf professionals who have evaluated my broken golf swing. These negative comments cause me no consternation. I am pleased to be a source of mirth to golf professionals, who seem like an overly serious bunch when I watch them on television. Any day I give another person a reason to smile or laugh is a great and blessed day. And I'm definitely heeding Mr. Palmer's advice, *"Don't quit your day job, Doctor."*

26

Million-Dollar Man

"You may not be able to change a situation, but with humor you can change your attitude about it."

Allen Klein

"Who sows virtue reaps honor."

Leonardo da Vinci

Humor: The quality of being amusing or comic, especially as expressed in literature or speech

Honor: High respect; great esteem; the quality of knowing and doing what is morally right

Cancer is indiscriminate and promiscuous. It strikes people without regard to socioeconomic status, education, title, gender, ethnicity, religion, or geographic location. Cancer doesn't care if you are a hard-working farmer, a housewife putting in twelve-plus-hour days raising a family, a student, a mechanic, a teacher, or a high-level executive at a big corporation. Cancer quite frankly doesn't give a damn how important you think you are.

It is my good fortune to meet and assist patients from highly variable and distinct backgrounds. I always enjoy learning about them, their families, and their lives. Surgical oncology is one of the specialties in medical practice that affords us a long-term relationship with our patients. The surgical operations I performed, along with multidisciplinary care, has successfully eradicated or controlled my patients' cancer in many cases. I have been seeing some patients in follow-up for more than fifteen or even twenty years. They have gone from asking about my kids' schoolwork and soccer teams to looking at photos of my kids' young children. A few weeks ago one of these patients commented that she was amazed to be seeing pictures of my grandkids. I replied, "Yeah, unbelievable isn't it? I'm way too young, don't you think?" She snorted and politely refrained from commenting on my age but corrected me by stating she meant she was happy to be alive for so many years after a diagnosis of stage IV cancer spread to her liver.

Some years ago I met a new patient referred to me by the medical oncologist who was treating him for six liver metastases from colorectal cancer. This particularly jolly, congenial, and animated gentleman was accompanied by his wife and three adult daughters at the initial clinic visit. When I walked in and introduced myself, he enthusiastically shook my hand and with a warm smile said, "I hope you can help me, Doc."

The patient had undergone removal of the primary tumor in his colon approximately nine months earlier. He was diagnosed with stage IV cancer because the adenocarcinoma had metastasized to lymph nodes near his colon and to his liver. He received six cycles, three months, of chemotherapy initially and the liver tumors had shrunk. After three more months of chemotherapy the tumors were stable, with no further reduction in size. When he came to see me his CT scan showed no evidence of tumor in any other location.

A part of any complete medical evaluation includes asking about a patient's occupation, activities, hobbies, and social habits. The last of these includes history of alcohol consumption, smoking cigarettes or other forms of tobacco, and any so-called recreational drug use. My patient was not a smoker, denied any illicit drug use, and told me he liked an occasional glass of wine or martini with dinner. We ask the other questions to learn about exposure to any types of hazardous chemicals or materials and to assess the fitness of our patient. The man sitting in front of me was well dressed, not overweight, and looked as if he could go out and run a mile or two. When I asked what he did for a living, he quickly replied, "I am a professional silver-tongued devil!" Never one to be outdone by a humorous remark, I shot back, "Your tongue looks red to me, but what's left of your hair is silver." He laughed and said, "Touché! You and I are going to get along famously."

This silver-haired/tongued gentleman and I finished his medical history, and I performed an examination. We then reviewed the images of his liver and decided an operation was indicated. At this point he revealed his true identity. He informed me he was a senior pilot for a large commercial airline. I knew this was important information because any patient who is a professional pilot must undergo rigorous testing and physical examinations to maintain his or her Federal Aviation Administration certification to fly. He informed me he would need written statements from me after his operation to allow him to return to the cockpit. I had done this before for other patients, so I assured him I was prepared to provide all appropriate and necessary documentation and certification of his medical fitness to fly.

This patient always had a few surprises up his sleeve for me.

He jerked a thumb over his shoulder at his wife and daughters and asked, "Do you think I will survive all of this?" Before I could respond, he let me know he had a one-million-dollar life insurance policy and the four women in the room were wondering when they would collect. There were loud protestations and comments like, "Oh, Daddy! You are such a pain!" Red-faced and huffing, the ladies instructed me not to believe anything he said. They assured me they didn't want his money but instead wanted him to survive, bad mannered though he was. He chuckled, and I soon learned incessant teasing was commonplace in this family. To their credit, his wife and daughters gave as well as they received, so there was always interesting and witty repartee among this group.

I scheduled the pilot for an operation a few weeks later. An intraoperative ultrasound demonstrated all six of his liver tumors were in the right lobe of his liver. We do not know why tumors metastasize in the occasionally odd but fortuitous pattern as they had in this man. It was possible to perform a straightforward right-liver-lobe resection and the procedure went without a hitch. There were no issues during his hospital stay and he was on a trajectory to recover well. About the third or fourth postoperative day I stopped by his room for a visit and found him alone. He informed me his wife and daughters had gone downstairs to grab a bite to eat. I pulled up a chair and sat next to his bed and asked, "How long have you been flying?" This simple question led to a lengthy and fascinating answer.

My patient confessed to being a graduate of the United States Naval Academy in Annapolis, Maryland. After graduation, he had gone to naval flight school and qualified to fly fighter jets. Growing up around my grandfather and his two brothers who had fought in World War II, I am a military-history aficionado and I frequently read books about military campaigns. I asked my patient to tell me more and learned he had piloted F-4 Phantoms off an aircraft carrier during the Vietnam War. He had flown numerous ground-support missions and combat sorties over two tours of duty. I asked—thoughtlessly, I realize in retrospect—if he had been involved in any dogfights with enemy MiGs. This usually jocular man became suddenly somber. He replied, "Affirmative. Two combat kills." He quietly added, "I don't talk about it much. It means somebody is dying up there. And I lost several friends and members of my air-combat squadron during the war." Recognizing it was time to change the subject but still enthralled to be sitting with a naval fighter pilot, I asked him to describe what it was like to take off and land on an aircraft carrier. His laugh returned immediately, "That is quite an experience." He went on to describe the hours of practice and the adrenaline rush associated with landing a jet on the deck. He provided an analogy and a description I will never forget: he said when approaching a carrier at a distance it looks like a postage stamp pitching and bobbing on the waves. He then described the controlled panic of a night landing in heavy seas and remarked comically, "It really tests your underarm deodorant."

About this time, the patient's wife and daughters returned, and he informed them we had been talking about his naval flight career. This induced eye rolling and comments from the four females in the room. The merciless taunting resumed, and I knew I had the help of these ladies in goading my patient into a rapid recovery.

The pilot continued to surprise me with tidbits of information. During his first postoperative clinic visit we discussed the necessary documentation to allow him to return to his airline. He noted that he wanted to resume working the following week. I informed him that would be too early to be flying an airplane. He admitted he was one of the senior captains charged with flight-simulator and safety training for his airline. He explained he would be on the ground, sitting at a console, and providing information and feedback to fellow pilots. He had no plans to return to the cockpit for at least three months post-op to assure he was ready to assume flight responsibilities. Satisfied, I replied I had no concerns as long as there was no heavy lifting or strenuous activity related to his duties. Laughing, he let me know there was no physical labor involved and his job was essentially "to scare the living daylights" out of fellow pilots by making sure they were prepared for all kinds of emergency ground and in-flight situations. I could envision this man with his wicked sense of humor deriving considerable pleasure out of tormenting his colleagues. I would learn that I was correct.

I followed the pilot for the next three years with follow-up visits. His blood tests were normal, his liver regenerated quickly to a regular volume, and his CT scans gloriously showed no evidence of recurrent metastatic disease. At every appointment his wife and three daughters were in the examination room with us. After I reported the good news, he invariably turned to them and let them know they would just have to wait for their million dollars. This produced immediate protestation and verbal jousting. He clearly knew how to push their buttons.

Midway through the fourth year of our routine visits I mentioned as an aside that I would be in his home city the following month to attend a surgical meeting. The patient asked if I would be interested in coming to his airline's flight-simulator facility. He indicated—a little too eagerly, I later realized—he would be happy to show me how they trained and tested pilots. I jumped at this opportunity, and on a Saturday morning I reported slightly early for our 9 a.m. appointment. He gave me a tour of the facility and introduced me to several of the people and the pilots working there. He then shepherded me into a Boeing 737 full-motion flight simulator. This was a large rectangular box sitting atop the heavy hydraulic pistons positioned around it. He informed me instructors could program the simulator to create the illusion of flying or landing in rough weather. He sat in the pilot's seat and told me to strap in to the co-pilot position. I held on to the yoke as we simulated a takeoff. After a few minutes he nonchalantly said, "Go ahead, make a few turns." I was thrilled to be flying this simulated aircraft and I completed a few meandering, simple maneuvers. He indicated it was time to "return to the runway" and showed me the checklist and steps involved in landing a commercial airliner. We came in smoothly and uneventfully, and he looked at me and said, "Voilà! That's how it's done." He got up and said, "Sit tight, Doc. I'll be right back."

He lied. He went out the door, and I sat waiting for about thirty seconds. Suddenly, the cockpit went dark; the virtual airplane windshield was black and I heard what sounded like rain pelting against the glass. Not possible—the simulator was indoors, wasn't it? The million-dollar man's preternaturally calm voice came from a speaker above my head. "Your pilot has just suffered a major medical problem and is incapacitated and unable to assist you. You are landing the plane alone at night in inclement weather. Good luck." *Is he serious?* The whole cabin started bucking like a bronco being spurred by a cowboy at the rodeo. I understood immediately why he had made me strap in because I would have been tossed around like an old T-shirt in a dryer had I not been secured to the seat. I looked at the altimeter as he instructed and saw the plane was at four thousand feet and descending. A monotonic female voice came over the cockpit radio and informed me my angle of approach was too low. Holding on to the yoke with a one-handed death grip, I began reducing air speed with the thrust levers as I had seen the pilot do. At the same time I applied the rudder pedals and flaps in an attempt to bring the plane in for a landing. After several minutes of bone-rattling shaking by the simulator, I suddenly saw the display of airstrip lights through the windshield and made corrections to line up on the runway. Each time I corrected, the whole box would shake violently as a simulated crosswind pushed me off course. *Thanks for that!* The female voice commented several more times on my low landing angle. I wanted to scream at her, "You are not helping!" I restrained myself and concentrated. I am not a pilot, and I have never flown an airplane, but I admit that at that moment I was completely immersed in trying to land this ultimate model airplane safely.

I managed to bring the aircraft in for a bumpy landing. After applying the brakes and bringing the plane to a halt, admittedly past the end of the simulated runway, my patient's laughter emanated from the loudspeaker over my head. "What did you think of that, Doc?" His obvious mirth and glee at my rapid heart and respiratory rate were not humorous to me. He opened the door grinning and said, "Hey, you look a little sweaty." Thanks for the statement of the obvious. I was perspiring like I had just run three miles on a hot Texas summer afternoon. I gained a great deal of respect for pilots that day. I also chided the million-dollar man with some choice words as we walked out, which did nothing but induce more chortling. He informed me several pilots had been in the control room watching, and on their behalf he thanked me for giving them a great show. You're welcome, always happy to provide some free entertainment.

Cancer is cancer and can rear its ugly head at any time. Almost five years after this gentleman's liver resection, his previously normal serum tumor marker for colorectal cancer was now elevated. His CT scan showed no tumors in his lungs, liver, or lymph nodes. However, there was a nodule in his right lower abdomen that had not been present before. This was the only abnormality I could detect on the scan. I suspected that this represented the proverbial tip of the iceberg and he likely had a situation called peritoneal carcinomatosis. This means tumor nodules spread throughout the belly cavity have implanted and are growing on the surface of organs in the abdomen and pelvis. Ironically, this was the first visit where only he and his wife were present because his daughters had all assumed he was fine and they no longer needed to come. I reviewed all of the images and test results with the pilot and his wife and shared my concern that this solitary nodule could represent a diffuse return of cancer throughout his abdominal cavity. He asked if I was sure of this and I informed him I was not. Nonetheless, I mentioned while I could remove this tumor, a case could be made to consider chemotherapy first. After a lengthy discussion of the rationale and pros and cons, he nodded and conceded it made sense to him to proceed with chemotherapy.

I called his medical oncologist, who was as disappointed as I upon learning the pilot's cancer had recurred. The oncologist initiated chemotherapy the next week, and I saw the pilot back three months later. His serum tumor marker had been reduced significantly and the tumor nodule was half the size it had been on previous scans. The patient looked at me and said, "Let's take it out." A very matter of fact, direct statement. I expressed hesitation but he noted it was the only spot detected on images, and he wanted to know if there was anything else hiding in his peritoneal cavity. I agreed to perform a laparoscopic exploration of his abdomen during surgery, but informed him this minimalist approach might be somewhat difficult because he had undergone a previous open-colon resection and a subsequent open-liver resection. Some patients after such operations have lots of scar tissue throughout the belly cavity. I mentioned I might be forced to make another open incision to get a good look at all areas. Undaunted, he readily agreed and we scheduled the operation for two weeks later.

Thankfully, he was one of the patients we occasionally see who forms very little scar tissue following abdominal surgery. I was able to get a thorough look at all areas of his peritoneal cavity using the laparoscope. I immediately found the tumor at the tip of the omentum, an apron of fatty tissue, lying in his right lower abdomen. It was a simple and straightforward matter to remove this small piece of fatty tissue and send it for pathological evaluation. Our pathologist froze the tumor, viewed it under the microscope and confirmed it was metastatic colon cancer. I looked at all of my patient's large and small intestine, the liver, and his stomach, and I even performed a laparoscopic ultrasound of the liver. I could find no additional tumor nodules. I next instilled a liter of sterile saline into his belly cavity through the laparoscopic ports. This is called peritoneal washing. I aspirated all of this fluid out into a canister and sent it to our cytopathologist to assess for the presence of malignant cells. I completed the operation and closed the small laparoscopic incisions.

When I checked on my patient in the recovery room two hours later, he was awake and alert and, as usual, smiling. His wife and three daughters were there at his bedside, the usual jibes being traded among them. As I walked up he shouted loudly enough for most of the patients and staff in the recovery room to hear, "I'm still here and they still don't get their million dollars!" I loved this guy. He was a naval aviator, a combat veteran, an airline pilot with thousands of hours of experience, and a real clown prince!

The cytopathology report revealed no evidence of additional malignant cells in the peritoneal cavity, a very bizarre situation. I had never before seen a single implant of colorectal cancer like this. Generally, when cancer occurs in the peritoneal cavity it is diffuse and scattered everywhere. We presented this gentleman's findings at a multidisciplinary tumor board and because his primary tumor responded and shrank with three months of chemotherapy, it was recommended he receive three more months of such treatment. This very reasonable and thoughtful gentleman understood the rationale and agreed to proceed. He completed his chemotherapy without difficulty or problem.

We resumed his follow-up routine. I saw him every four months for the next three years. At a visit into his fourth year of follow-up after the second operation I had performed, I pulled up his lab results, and once again his serum tumor marker was elevated. This time it was much higher than it had been previously. I opened his CT images on the computer and saw that the monster had returned with a vengeance. Now, there were several dozen new lung metastases and enlarged lymph nodes in his chest and along the aorta and inferior vena cava behind his intestines.

I walked forlornly into the examination room shaking my head. The pilot and his family immediately understood. Before I said anything, he turned and grasped his wife's hand and told her he had expected bad news because he had not been feeling completely normal. I have heard many patients make similar statements when they are diagnosed with seemingly asymptomatic cancer. Even though the patients don't have any specific symptoms, they somehow sense or know their cancer has recurred. The patient, his wife, and daughters maintained a stoic facade as we discussed the findings and treatment options. I explained this was not a situation we could treat with surgery or any type of radiation therapy. He nodded, understanding, and from the examination room I called his medical oncologist. We discussed this aggressive, albeit somewhat late pattern of recurrence. This patient had already had two types of standard chemotherapy regimens for stage IV colorectal cancer. We weighed numerous options and the patient decided after seeing his medical oncologist the next week to enroll in a clinical trial.

Clinical trials are critical to study new drugs, combinations of agents, or alternative approaches to treat a variety of cancer types. By definition, many of the agents used in clinical trials are new and do not have long-term survival results or response rates. This is a critical mechanism to study new therapies as we continuously seek better treatments to produce better survival rates, and hopefully better quality of life for our patients.

Unfortunately, the pilot's cancer did not respond after he received a study drug for almost three months. He went from being asymptomatic, looking fit and normal, to a haggard, sallow, and drawn appearance. When I saw him, his wife, and daughters in the office and informed them of the results, he nodded quietly and said, "I'm through." He told me he wanted no more chemotherapy side effects, and he was content with the additional decade of life he had already gained through two operations and chemotherapy. This was the only time I saw his wife and daughters weep. They did so quietly and with dignity. I sat with the pilot and his family for another thirty minutes, providing what comfort I could and answering tough questions on what to expect as the cancer progressed. I asked him to call me and keep me updated on how he was feeling and getting along. He did call twice in the next two months, but the third call I received was from his wife to report that he had died peacefully at home surrounded by his family.

I was invited to his funeral the next week but was unable to attend because I had two major liver operations already scheduled that day. I later learned from one of his daughters he had been buried with full military honors, including a flyover by U.S. Navy F/A-18 Hornets from a nearby naval air station. She told me when flying over the cemetery; one plane pulled up vertically and peeled off from the others to signify a missing-man formation. She informed me the church and the funeral service had been packed with hundreds of people who celebrated the life and vitality of the pilot.

Our patients are amazing people. All of them. They are remarkable and they come with occasionally unexpected backgrounds; some are simple salt-of-the earth types, others have incredible past and current occupations or skills and interesting histories and stories to tell. The pilot, the million-dollar man, embodied two virtues I value highly, honor and humor. Two capital *H* attributes of great worth, I believe. I respect and salute him, and all cancer patients.

27

Great Case

Commitment: The state or quality of being dedicated to a cause, activity, or goal

Humans have different coping mechanisms to deal with stress, fatigue, emotional overload, and repetitive actions in our daily lives. Health-care providers, like people in many other professions, must manage interpersonal interactions and pressure routinely. Sadly, a common stress-minimization method I have noticed among surgeons is actually a bit dehumanizing. The specific coping technique I have witnessed repeatedly ever since I was a medical student is to refer to a patient by the body part of surgical interest rather than the patient's name. This is ironic because our patients grant us surgeons ultimate trust and access, which is a highly personal experience.

A few examples: During my general-surgery rotation as a third-year medical student, our team of medical students and junior residents began each morning long before the sun rose. Our first daily job, before 6 a.m., was to collect all of the requisite information on vital signs and laboratory data from the hospitalized surgical patients. We would then tag along behind the chief surgical resident as he or she went from room to room to evaluate and examine the inpatients before beginning the day's schedule of operations. If asked, we students were expected to recite from memory a specific lab value, maximum temperature, or urine output from the previous shift. It was commonplace for the chief resident to ask, "How's the gallbladder in forty-three doing?" or "What's the drain output from the pancreas in ICU?" As we completed rounds, the residents would begin discussing the operations to be performed: "I'm doing the aorta today, are you doing the right colon?" and "Did you remember to consent the hernia?"

What exactly is the hernia consenting to?

It was rare to hear one of the surgery residents state correctly and deferentially, "I am going to perform the gastric resection on Mr. Smith today. Why don't you help Dr. Jones remove the gallbladder from Mrs. Thomas?" This depersonalization of patients continued throughout my surgical residency, surgical oncology fellowship, and into the early years of my academic career. As a senior and chief resident I drove the younger residents mad by insisting they identify patients by their name, not by a diseased or damaged organ like "the bleeding esophagus," "the pancreatic cancer," or "the cirrhotic liver." However, it took me a few years to attain a level of seniority as an academic surgeon before I felt comfortable addressing this vexation with my peers and colleagues. Now when I politely correct them after they refer to a patient as "the stomach" or some other anatomical site, I am invariably met with frosty glares, lack of comprehension, or a shake of the head.

That's right, I'm at it again.

An important reality of modern cancer care is the still-crucial role surgical treatment plays in improving patients' probability of long-term survival. For many organ-based solid cancers, surgical removal of the primary tumor, affected regional lymph nodes, and (in specific cancer types and instances), metastatic deposits of tumor continues to provide patients the best chance of beating their disease. This in no way is meant to minimize the role of chemotherapy, radiation therapy, immunotherapy, targeted therapies, or other multidisciplinary approaches. The team approach to treating cancer is clearly beneficial to patients and improves their odds of survival. Surgery is still dominant, however, when it comes to removing large or aggressive cancers.

This reality leads to another misdirected euphemism among surgical trainees and staff surgeons: their wonderment over an unusual, difficult, or particularly grueling and technically demanding operation. Residents or fellows will regale others in their program with a remark like "Wow, the liver I did yesterday was a great case!" or "I'm doing a tough bile duct with a vein resection with Curley today. It's going to be a great case!" Most surgeons like doing challenging, big operations. Frankly, for me, the advanced, exacting surgical methods and the variety of sites involved was a major draw to a career in surgical oncology. Performing routine, mundane procedures is fine, but surgeons get a little amped up at the prospect of a "great case." However, I fear we forget too commonly the great case is a really big, frightening prospect for the patient who is unknowingly being dehumanized.

Early in my career after completing my surgical oncology–fellowship training, a patient was referred to me because he had a large right-colon cancer. His tumor was easily palpable through the abdominal wall. The patient was a thin gentleman in his mid-forties who had lost almost twenty pounds over the preceding three months. He had not intended to lose weight and had not been dieting. The gastroenterologist who referred the patient to me had performed a colonoscopy and a CT scan that revealed a large mass in the colon just beneath the liver.

Usually, if a colon cancer is related to weight loss it is advanced or metastatic to other organs. I looked at this gentleman's CT scan and saw there was no evidence of enlarged lymph nodes or any tumors in the liver, peritoneal cavity, or lungs. I also noticed the tumor was larger than a cantaloupe and was abutting the duodenum (the first part of the small intestine) and the head of his pancreas. The small intestine is critical to absorb nutrients from the food we eat while the colon is involved in conserving water and storing and excreting waste products. I asked the patient if he was having pain related to the cancer and he replied he was not. But when I asked if he was having trouble eating he admitted he felt full after only a few bites of food. He paused, and as an afterthought reported he avoided eating because with even a small meal or snack he felt queasy, and on several occasions had vomited food and some blood.

Vomiting blood was a red flag. Patients with colon cancer may notice blood in their bowel movements, but bloody emesis is not common. I asked one of my gastroenterology colleagues to perform an upper-gastrointestinal endoscopy to look into his esophagus, stomach, and duodenum. This revealed his colon cancer had grown into a portion of the duodenum. A biopsy confirmed colon cancer was present near the ampulla of Vater, the location where the bile duct and pancreatic duct drain from the liver and pancreas, respectively, into the duodenum.

As I looked at the images from the endoscope, I exhaled with a low-volume whistle. This was going to be a big operation, the proverbial great case. I met with the patient and his family and explained that his colon cancer had grown into the first part of his small intestine and was also involving the head of his pancreas. With anatomical diagrams and drawings I described the operation I proposed. This would involve a surgical tour de force, an en bloc (everything taken out together in one large specimen) extended right hemicolectomy and pancreaticoduodenectomy. All told, the operation would remove a few inches of the terminal ileum (the last part of the small intestine where it joins into the right colon), the entire right colon and most of the transverse colon, the distal (last) portion of the stomach, the entire duodenum, the head of the pancreas, the gallbladder and a portion of the common bile duct, and the proximal jejunum for a few inches past where the duodenum joins the jejunum at the ligament of Treitz. (Sorry for all the anatomy terminology.)

I took a good thirty minutes detailing the operation and I emphasized the implications of four anastomoses, or surgical connections, I would perform. The remaining pancreas and the common bile duct would each need to be reattached to the small intestine, the stomach would need to be sutured to the small intestine so ingested food could exit from the stomach into the intestine to be absorbed, and the transected end of the ileum would need to be attached to the remaining colon.

The surgical resident and fellow in the clinic room with me were as wide-eyed as the patient and his family. I explained that the operation would be a large-magnitude procedure, but I believed it provided him the best chance to remove the malignant tumor completely and give him hope for a reasonable period of survival.

Everyone knows the saying about hindsight, and my remarks to the patient were more than prophetic. Despite his weight loss, the gentleman was nutritionally still in good condition. The next week we performed the operation, which required more than seven hours from incision to final skin suture. The patient was

stable throughout the procedure and the morning after his operation he was alert and optimistic. He had a drain tube protrud-
ing from his abdomen to watch for a leak from the pancreatic
anastomosis to the small intestine. And because I was concerned
about his nutritional status with the combination of weight loss
and a complex, major resection a second tube was placed directly
into his small intestine (a procedure called a feeding jejunos-
tomy) to allow us to begin feedings. Surprisingly, we never had
to use it. His bowel function returned within forty-eight hours,
and we allowed him to begin drinking small amounts of fluids
gingerly. He breezed through a liquid diet and by day four was
eating solid food, wolfing it down, and asking for more. My suspi-
cion that his family was providing him with contraband fast food
was confirmed when I walked into his hospital room on day six to
find hamburgers and french fries being held or chewed and swal-
lowed rapidly by all. Guilty facial expressions were replaced by
smiles and laughter when I said, "What the hell—you didn't bring
me one?"

My patient remained hospitalized for an additional two days,
frankly more as treatment for my anxiety rather than as medical
necessity, and before he was discharged, both his drain and feeding tube were removed. He was eating well, and his bowels were
functioning well. I saw him back in the office the following week.
He had gained three pounds and was pleased with the surgical
results. I reviewed his extensive pathology report with the entire
family. The examining pathologist had indicated that the large
cancer arising from his colon had indeed invaded directly into the
duodenum and the head of his pancreas. More than sixty lymph
nodes had been removed during the operation, and remarkably
there had been no evidence of cancer in any of them. All resection margins were negative by several centimeters. The final
analysis: he had a locally advanced cancer invading into adjacent

organs but that had not metastasized to lymph nodes or to any other organ.

The following week I presented my patient's findings at a multidisciplinary tumor conference. As I walked in, I overheard my fellow talking to other surgical fellows and residents. He exclaimed, "What a great case. The colon-Whipple did great!" At that moment, he caught my eye and quickly corrected course knowing what remark I would make otherwise. He amended his comments and told his colleagues the patient with a right-colon cancer locally invading adjacent organs had recovered very well from his right colon resection-pancreaticoduodenectomy (Whipple) procedure.

Uh-huh. A close call for the fellow. Don't make me come over there and talk to you about referring to patients by their body parts.

My colleagues in medical oncology could not find a data-based reason to administer chemotherapy treatment to improve this gentleman's prognosis. Admittedly, at the time we did not have many of the drugs we now have available for locally advanced or invasive colorectal cancer. These days, the patient would likely receive preoperative chemotherapy to try to reduce the size of the tumor. But at the time, I called my patient with the recommendation we simply follow him closely and we would intervene with additional therapies if and when his cancer recurred.

I had that conversation with my patient twenty-three years ago. He is alive, vibrant, and active, and his cancer has never recurred. He exemplifies the importance of being committed to surgical-technique excellence when operating on patients with cancer. Complete surgical removal with negative margins is a goal we strive for in every patient. However, negative margins are not always possible because we may discover during an operation that cancer is invading vital sites we cannot remove without doing irreparable or life-threatening damage to the patient. This is why we frequently decide not to perform an operation when preoperative scans reveal tumor growing into or abutting critical structures we cannot remove or replace. In those situations our colleagues often give preoperative chemotherapy or a combination of chemotherapy and radiation therapy to shrink the tumor so we can hopefully perform a complete resection at a subsequent date.

My patient's success story is not unique. It is well known that some types of cancer tend to invade locally into structures or organs around them, and in a subset of patients when complete surgical removal of all cancer is possible, long-term survival may result. However, a major surgical procedure has implications on a patient's lifestyle, functions, body image, and nutrition. The patient may have a successful cancer operation but be forced to live with stomas, deformities, or other disabilities. Every now and then, we encounter a patient like mine who underwent an extensive operation and recovered well. He is thriving, and except for a long scar on his abdomen, you would never know he was a cancer survivor.

This represents a great result after a great case. I'm still working on the objectification problem, however. A couple of years ago I was planning to remove a malignant tumor in the left liver lobe of a very amiable gentleman. During the operation, I recognized that the malignant tumor was invading into the diaphragm. The surgical resident and I opened the diaphragm, planning to remove a small piece of this muscle attached to the tumor and then close the defect. I had encountered this situation dozens of times previously. Instead, we found the tumor had grown through the diaphragm and was attached to the right ventricle of the heart. That was a novel situation; I hadn't seen this problem before.

I am fortunate to work now at an institution with a renowned cardiothoracic-surgery center. I called over to the heart operating rooms, had two cardiothoracic surgeons come join me, and within twenty minutes my patient was on full cardiopulmonary bypass. The cardiac surgeons removed a piece of the apex of the right ventricle stuck to the liver tumor, I completed the liver resection, they closed the hole in his heart, and the patient came off the bypass smoothly. All of our margins, including the heart, were tumor-free, and the patient walked out of the hospital the following week.

A few days after this remarkable procedure, I encountered one of the cardiac surgeons who had assisted me. He was sitting in the surgeons' lounge waiting for his next operation to begin. I remarked, "You know, Mr. So and So is recovering really well. Amazing! Thanks for your help."

He looked at me with a puzzled expression, and suddenly, the light bulb went on.

"Oh, the liver-heart guy. Yeah, great case."

Long sigh. Change is usually not easy or fast.

My mission continues.

28

Surf's Up

"Contentment is the only real wealth."

Alfred Nobel

Contentment: A state of happiness and satisfaction

At the pinnacle of its power and influence, the Roman Empire extended across large portions of Europe, Western Asia, and Northern Africa. To maintain peace and to display authority and prosperity, the leaders of Rome designated many days as celebrations or "holy days" to give thanks to a variety of gods in the pre-Christian era. Holy days became holidays in modern parlance. There were almost 140 identified days or periods for feasting and festival in the Julian calendar. The Roman population apparently liked a good party, causing the Emperors of Rome to go to the trouble and expense of sponsoring bloody battles at the Colosseum, chariot races at the Circus Maximus, and festive parades and performances.

Assigning more than one-third of the calendar year for feast and folly may be one factor that led to the decline of the Roman

Empire. The lack of productive and useful work by celebrating citizens certainly could not have helped maintain the empire. Political corruption, abuse of power, declining moral values, expansion into far-reaching territories, and excessive spending on public works and military campaigns also contributed to the end of the empire.

Doesn't history repeat itself? One thing can be said about the modern United States; we are not to be outdone by the Roman Empire. We have more than 2,300 recognized or declared holidays or observances. These special celebrations may last a day, a few days, a week, or a month. In fairness, very few of our sanctioned holidays actually are a day off from usual work and other banal duties. Like our ancient Roman brethren, though, we do expect a spectacle on a few special days. What would the Fourth of July be without rousing marching bands or extravagant, brilliant, exploding fireworks? What is Thanksgiving without turkey-based (or basted turkey) gluttony, parades, and televised football games? Why observe Labor Day if we don't relax from our labors with a barbecue and a gathering of family and friends? Memorial Day would not be memorable without speeches, parades, and American flags displayed on the graves of American soldiers during somber ceremonies across the nation.

Paradoxically, the majority of special days, weeks, or months in America pass without fanfare or much notice. Did you save your unwanted, untouched, hardened holiday fruitcake and fling it across your yard on January 3 to commemorate National Fruitcake Toss Day? Or heave it over the backyard fence as a special Happy New Year gift for your neighbors? You know, the folks with the teenagers who like to play really loud music. At 2:30 a.m. On week nights. How much money did you spend hosting an exhilarating festival at your home on July 19 for National Hot Dog Day, and did you double down with an even bigger party on September

9 for National Weiner Schnitzel Day? Tell me you displayed red, white, and green decorations and made a nice marinara sauce on February 13 for National Tortellini Day. Was your family driven into a sugar-fueled frenzy on May 19 after eating all of the chocolate cake they wanted to honor National Devil's Food Cake Day?

What are your plans for the entire month of October, appointed as National Toilet Tank Repair Month? Should we be concerned that toilet-tank repair requires an entire month for adequate homage? Does excessive flushing during the summer months lead to tired tanks in need of service to prepare for the winter holiday season? And what happens if the toilet bowl breaks? Must we wait for a special month to seal or replace a cracked and leaking crapper? My grandfather, my father's father, was a union plumber his entire adult life. Is the plumbing lobby in Washington, D.C., responsible for acquiring official recognition for an entire month to extol the virtues of a properly functioning toilet tank? I must wonder if money is being privately passed under the bowl in the privy.

If you play your cards right, you can spend any given week in daily blissful celebration. I'll give you an example of how to make big plans for the first week of June. On June 1, as an important public-safety exercise, you can teach a class at your place of employment in honor of National Heimlich Maneuver Day. It's critical for people to know the proper administration of the Heimlich maneuver. Convince your boss to take the entire office out to lunch, just in case an actual food-induced airway obstruction occurs. Parenthetically, you will be sock- and shoeless during your Heimlich demonstrations because June 1 is also National Go Barefoot Day. No worries if you exhaust yourself teaching the maneuver because June 2 is National Leave the Office Early Day. Thankfully, there is no official code stating how early one can leave, so why not take off after a 9:30 a.m. coffee break? The week just keeps getting better; June 3 is National Repeat Day, so you'll leave work early again. Well-rested and invigorated by the holiday mood, identify an older unmarried woman on June 4 and ask her to join you at a local pub to enjoy a fine brandy to celebrate both National Old Maids' Day and National Cognac Day. In high spirits after a few snifters of brandy, you may not get much accomplished at your job on June 5 as you enjoy National Moonshine Day. You know moonshine is illegal, right? But it still has its own official national day. Is America great or what? The moonshine will have you relaxed, loose, and ready to demonstrate manual dexterity on June 6 for National Yo-Yo Day. The week will end on a high note, especially if you are a card-carrying chocoholic, because on June 7 you can pound down your own half gallon to revel on National Chocolate Ice Cream Day. Great week! And it works for every other week, too, if you apply your sanctioned and recognized holidays to full advantage.

Many types of cancer are emphasized during specific months of the year. Nearly every month is designated to raise awareness for one or more cancers. This is intended to remind Americans of the importance of prevention, screening, early diagnosis, and research to improve treatments, survival rates, and quality-of-life outcomes for a particular cancer. For example, April is Testicular Cancer Awareness Month and it includes the graphically named Get a Grip campaign. Let's be gentle with the grip. Can we agree on that?

A patient of mine I saw recently caused me to think about October.

October is National Breast Cancer Awareness Month, and it is one of the most highly visible and publicized awareness months assigned to a specific cancer diagnosis. It is great fun for me to watch very large men wearing tight uniforms, heavy pads, and football helmets crash into one another while wearing pink shoes, pink wristbands, and pink towels. Smash-mouth, grind-out-a-few-yards running plays seem a little less ferocious when the 310-pound pulling guard, the 230-pound running back he leads into the six-hole, and the 250-pound outside linebacker he collides with are all wearing bright pink cleats. Even the officials get into the act by wearing pink armbands and blowing pink whistles. While it may seem enigmatic to see football players prancing in pink, it actually makes perfect sense.

All of us, including professional athletes, have a mother. Often a sideline television camera will capture a close-up of a football player who just completed a great play as he looks into the camera, waving and says, "Hi Mom!" Despite our many advances in cancer research and therapeutics, breast cancer is still one of the three most common causes of cancer-related deaths in women in America. (The other two are lung and colorectal cancer.) It is estimated that approximately one in eight American women will develop breast cancer during their lifetime. As a shocking news flash to the guys, breast cancer can occur, rarely, in men. It's not just the ladies who are at risk, Lads. Unlike some deep body cavity cancers, this tumor is easier to detect with routine screening examinations. Mammography and ultrasound administered regularly can diagnose small, early-stage breast cancers and save thousands of lives. That's why biannual screening mammography in individuals with no family history of breast cancer is currently recommended to begin at age fifty.

The patient who induced me to muse about pink-footed football players is an outstanding young woman. When I met her she was an executive at a large firm in a major American urban center. Shortly after turning thirty, she noticed a painless lump in her breast. She astutely and immediately sought medical care and a mammogram confirmed the presence of a mass that was potentially malignant.

This young lady had no family history of breast or any other kind of cancer. She was referred to a breast surgical specialist who performed a detailed examination and palpated several enlarged lymph nodes under her arm, an anatomic area called the axilla. An ultrasound-guided biopsy of the breast tumor and enlarged lymph nodes confirmed infiltrating ductal carcinoma of the breast with metastasis to the regional lymph nodes. Additional special stains of her biopsy slides revealed her tumor expressed estrogen and progesterone receptors and was positive for human epidermal growth factor receptor 2 (HER2). The presence of estrogen or progesterone receptors in breast cancer has been known for several decades to be useful information guiding long-term delivery of anti-estrogen drugs to help control and prevent recurrence of this tumor. The additional indication of overexpression of HER2 on the surface of the cancer cells is a more recent discovery. HER2 expression is one example of a modern molecular-profiling study that is now routinely performed to assess treatment options for patients with advanced malignant disease. The presence of this receptor on the surface of breast-cancer cells allows use of a specific drug, a monoclonal antibody called trastuzumab, in combination with other chemotherapy drugs to improve the killing of the malignant breast-cancer cells throughout the body. Conversely, the absence of these three receptors in breast cancer, so called triple-negative breast cancer, portends a more aggressive cancer and indicates that the use of anti-estrogen or trastuzumab therapy will not be helpful.

The patient was referred to a medical oncologist who found all metastatic evaluation studies, including a positron emission tomography (PET) scan and CT scans of the brain, chest, abdomen, and pelvis were negative except for a single 2.5-centimeter tumor in the right lobe of her liver. This tumor had the appearance of a possible metastasis on the CT scan, and had a high

uptake of the radiolabeled glucose molecules used on the PET
scan, which was also worrisome as a possible malignant lesion. An
interventional radiologist performed a biopsy of the liver tumor.
The presence of stage IV breast cancer with a solitary liver metastasis was established.

She received three months of systemic intravenous chemotherapy including trastuzumab, and the tumor in the upper, outer
quadrant of her breast and the lymph nodes shrank markedly.
Her liver tumor also decreased in volume by approximately one-
quarter. She underwent a breast-sparing operation removing the
malignant tumor and a surrounding zone of normal breast tissue
accompanied by removal of all of the lymph nodes in the armpit. The pathology studies confirmed her cancer showed a major
response to the chemotherapy, but there were still viable cancer
cells in the breast tumor and the lymph nodes. At this point, all
of the patient's malignant disease except for the single liver tumor
had been removed. That is when she contacted me.

Within ten minutes of meeting this highly intelligent, well-
educated, articulate young woman in the clinic, it was clear to me
she was focused and well informed. She had already read reports
from the surgical oncology literature describing the long-term survival probabilities of women who underwent surgical resection
of breast-cancer liver metastases. In addition to inquiring about
resection of her liver metastasis, she wanted to know if ablation
techniques, including radiofrequency or microwave thermal ablation, would be indicated in her. I had ordered a high resolution
CT scan of her abdomen the day before her visit with me, and I
pulled up the images on the computer screen in the examination
room.

Scrolling through the scans, I immediately realized ablation
techniques were not an option for her because the single tumor
was nestled between the anterior and posterior branch of her right

portal vein. The liver has both arterial and venous blood supply, and coursing along the hepatic-artery and portal-vein branches into the liver are large bile ducts. Performing thermal destruction of a tumor in that location would kill the tumor, but would also destroy major bile-duct branches and produce significant and dangerous injury to normal tissue. I showed the patient and her family the CT images and then used pictures and drawings of liver anatomy to explain why ablation was not appropriate. She replied with a nod and asked me to describe the operation needed to remove her liver metastasis. I believe it was a rhetorical question, more for her family than for her because as I described the anatomical rationale for performing a formal right hepatectomy removing approximately two-thirds of her liver, she again nodded her head while her family members gasped. The location of this single metastasis abutting the blood supply to the right lobe of the liver necessitated removal of the entire lobe to assure a tumor-free margin would be attained.

We had an approximately sixty-minute conversation about the potential benefits, alternatives, and risks of a major surgical procedure. The patient's family appeared rather frazzled, but she calmly announced at the end of our conversation that she was ready to proceed.

The next week I performed an uneventful right hepatectomy on this young lady. The procedure was completed in less than two hours with minimal blood loss, and she was awake, alert, and asking me questions in the recovery room within thirty minutes of finishing the operation. Generally after major liver resections, patients are hospitalized for five or six days. On the morning of her third postoperative day, she was fully dressed in her civilian clothes and reported that she was ready to go home. Her laboratory values and overall performance status confirmed she was ready to go, so discharge orders were dutifully written. I saw her back in the clinic a few days later, and we reviewed her pathology report. As with her primary breast cancer and axillary lymph nodes, there was evidence of a significant response to her chemotherapy regimen, but some viable cancer cells remained. The resection margins were clear.

While sitting in the room with the patient and her family, I called her medical oncologist and discussed the findings. We agreed in a real-time tumor board that she should receive additional chemotherapy and targeted therapy with trastuzumab. She returned home to her life, work, and ongoing chemotherapy treatment. After completing a total of six months of cytotoxic chemotherapy, she continued to receive infusions of the targeted agent. This monotherapy went on for another year, during which time I saw her every four months and happily reported blood tests and imaging studies showed she was cancer-free.

I've been seeing this patient twice a year now. She is more than five years out from her right-liver-lobe resection for metastatic breast cancer. I always saw her as a composed, reserved, decisive, professional individual. At her most recent visit things changed. When I walked into the room she was tanned and her hair had a sun-bleached appearance. Her usually serious demeanor was replaced by a wide smile and she rose from her chair and gave me a warm hug. She has never hugged me before. Laughing at my startled expression, she reported, "I decided it was time to enjoy life and lighten up." I wondered if she was performing a feat of mind reading because she preemptively stated, "I know you're going to say something about my tan. Don't worry, I'm using a good sunscreen." Melanoma prevention is important, too. And not just in May, during Melanoma Awareness Month.

She went on to surprise me further. She told me her cancer

diagnosis had initially driven her to do all she could to survive, but she realized she wasn't enjoying her life. A few weeks after my previous visit with her, she decided to quit her job and do something she had always dreamt of doing. Specifically, she wanted to learn how to surf. She moved to the West Coast and rented a small house near a famous surf beach. She sought out local surfers and instructors, bought a short board, and began to ride the waves every day. She pulled a portfolio out of her satchel and showed me series of pictures. The first few photos were of her in a wet suit standing nervously on a surf board in two-foot surf. The pictures progressed to a final shot taken three weeks earlier on the north shore of Maui with her clad in a bikini, grinning widely, and successfully riding a nine-foot wave, several feet above her head. I looked at her and said, "Cowabunga, Baby!"

She laughed heartily and assured me she did not plan to turn into a professional surf bum. She had started her own consulting business after realizing she was happy with a simpler, less-stressful life. She plans to continue her voyage, to become a better surfer, to live her life fully, to volunteer and help others, and to find reasons to enjoy every day. It sounded like a great plan to me. I complimented her on her decision and reported as an afterthought, "Oh yeah, all of your scans and blood tests are normal. Everything is looking great." That news earned me a second hug. She promised to keep me updated on her surfing adventures and I promised to enjoy living vicariously through her experiences.

Some people are overwhelmed by fear and apprehension after being diagnosed with a potentially life-threatening, chronic disease. Others, like this young lady, use the experience to redirect their lives and goals. I understand and empathize with both mind-sets, but I use stories like the one about my young surfer to encourage patients I see who are encumbered by anxiety and uncertainty that keep them from enjoying their daily lives. The surfer understands her breast cancer may recur, but she does not allow that knowledge to prey on her well-being and happiness. Life is uncertain and, frankly, none of us know how many days we have left to walk this earth. Every day should be embraced with joy and hopefulness.

Surf's up.

After all, every day is a holiday.

29

This Is Too Real

"My mission in life is not merely to survive, but to thrive; and to do so with some passion, some compassion, some humor, and some style."

Maya Angelou

Compassion: Sympathetic pity and concern for the sufferings or misfortunes of others

When we humans find ourselves in a new social setting with people we have not met or don't know well, there are certain unwritten but accepted rules of engagement. Unless you are attending a rally supporting your favorite candidate, it is generally not a good idea to open conversations with strangers with a discourse on politics. Similarly, if you are not in church, it may not be an opportune moment to initiate a conversation about religion. Instead, we choose socially accepted, banal, safe topics:

"Can you believe how hot it's been this month?"
"I had a foot of standing water in my back yard after all the rain we've been having."

"Do you think [name your favorite sports team here] will win
   this weekend?"
"What do you do for a living?"

The last is a very common inquiry when meeting an individual or group of people for the first time. It's a reasonably prudent
opener and usually leads to a set of nonthreatening and nonemo-
tional follow-up questions or comments, such as:

"Are there others in your family who do similar work?"
"How long have you been doing that?"
"Gee, that must be interesting."

But it's not so when I am asked the question. Until five or six
years ago, when someone queried about my vocation, I would
respond directly, "I am a surgical oncologist. I operate on patients
who have liver, pancreas, and gastrointestinal cancers."

I wish I had a video camera to record people's responses and
facial expressions after I gave my answer. Eyebrows would rise,
rapid blinking would occur, smiles would disappear, and weight
would be shifted from one foot to the other as the inquiring
individual processed this information. After quickly contemplat-
ing the implications of my professional activities, people would
cough affectedly and change the subject. Some would excuse
themselves reporting they had just seen a person across the
room they wanted to greet, allowing them to move rapidly away
from me, as if cancer were a communicable disease. And others would say something like, "Oh, that must be difficult. How
do you handle dealing with cancer patients and such an awful
disease?"

Currently, when new people I meet ask about my job I alert
them with, "Are you sure you want to know? Careful what you

wish for." Inevitably they are intrigued; I am pressed for an answer. Despite being forewarned, I still get the same responses.

It just makes it a little more fun for me.

After recovering from initially being surprised, many people tell me stories about their personal experiences with cancer. It is rare to meet an individual who has not been affected by cancer in a family member, friend, or colleague. Or the person may be a cancer survivor him- or herself. It is a pervasive disease and a topic that invokes an emotional response.

I recently spoke to a group of about seventy first-year medical students. Members of the faculty had been asked to talk with students about different career paths in medicine. I described my daily activities and then opened the floor to questions. The first one was another common question I'm asked: "What made you decide to become a cancer surgeon?"

I often startle people with my ardent response.

"It's personal for me. I hate cancer. I hate what it does to people and their families. When I was a junior surgical resident, one of my cousins, then an eighteen-year-old girl beginning her senior year in high school, was diagnosed with stage IV Ewing's sarcoma. She was treated in the university hospital where I was a resident. Over ten months I watched her endure terrible pain and horrific side effects from treatment. Her death was agonizing. I saw what the experience did to her and to my aunt and uncle, my parents, my cousins, and everyone who loved her. All these years later, I am still pissed off. It's just not right, and we have to do something to find better ways to understand, prevent, and treat cancer."

Somber silence. There's not much people can think to say after a monologue dripping with venom.

Sometimes people will ask how I deal with the angst and distress of patients who are diagnosed with a cancer I cannot treat surgically, or when their cancer recurs and metastasizes despite

all of our multidisciplinary treatments. My response is rooted in a
baseball analogy. The greatest hitters in baseball successfully get
a hit and find themselves on one of the four bases approximately
one-third of the time. This means they fail to get on base the
majority of their at bats. They may strike out, fly out, or ground
out to an infielder. Less effective hitters may have a success rate
of only one in four or one in five times at bat. If your batting average is lower than that, unless you are a pitcher, you will likely find
yourself shipped to a minor-league team. I go on to explain that
with many cancers our success rate with surgical and other treatments falls in range of the batting average of a middling-to-elite
major-league baseball player. For some cancers, our success rate
is much worse, and we need to work diligently to find better treatments or ship ourselves back into the basic science laboratories to
find something better to help people. Happily, for some cancers
we now have treatment-success averages that are unimaginable
for even the best major-league hitters. But we are still not anywhere close to batting a thousand.

Caring for cancer patients is not an easy job and can incite
intense emotions. A few years ago, I met a woman in her early
fifties who was astonished when she was diagnosed with stage IV
colorectal cancer. She had been a busy and healthy individual,
involved in numerous community and church activities and with
no medical problems. Along with her husband she was engaged
in raising two teenage children, who were soon to enter college.
She was feeling less energetic than usual, and had noticed a few
episodes of some bright-red blood mixed in with her bowel movements. A trip to her family physician was followed quickly by a
referral to a gastroenterologist. The gastroenterologist performed
a colonoscopy and discovered a circumferential but nonobstructing cancer in the left side of her colon. The gastroenterologist ordered a CT scan of her chest, abdomen, and pelvis to

evaluate her appropriately for the presence of any metastatic disease. Unfortunately the scans revealed five lemon-sized tumors in the right lobe of her liver.

The patient was immediately referred to a medical oncologist who began intravenous chemotherapy. He administered six cycles of chemotherapy, a two-day intravenous infusion every two weeks. He then referred the patient to me. This woman and her husband were well-educated professionals who had read extensively about her disease. They came prepared with several pages of questions, and I dutifully answered all of them. She was no longer bleeding from the primary tumor in the colon, and reviewing a new set of CT scans showed that the colon cancer, which had been readily evident on her initial scans, had decreased in size markedly. The five liver tumors were also smaller, but one tumor was very near the right portal vein and hepatic artery providing the blood supply to the right lobe of the liver. Another tumor was draped around the right hepatic vein. We had a long conversation about the sequence of surgical treatment, and I recommended we proceed with removal of the right lobe of her liver first. Her primary tumor had decreased in size and was causing no problems, and I was concerned that taking her off chemotherapy for two or three months while she recovered from a colon operation would allow the liver tumors to grow back to a potentially dangerous size. The patient and her family understood the rationale and agreed to proceed.

A surgical oncologist must assess the timing, sequence, and specific operation to perform in each individual patient diagnosed with stage IV colorectal cancer. Multidisciplinary cancer care is not a simple formula; each person should receive a customized treatment plan. In some patients, we are able to remove both the primary colorectal cancer and the liver metastases in a single operation. In others, the volume of liver removed combined with the potential extent of an oncological colon or rectal resection is deemed too much for a patient to tolerate physiologically. If a patient has a malignant tumor obstructing the colon or rectum, the priority is to remove the primary tumor, and the liver metastases are dealt with later. Often, patients receive chemotherapy first, before any surgical procedure, and if the liver metastases are a greater risk than the primary tumor, the liver resection is completed before a colorectal surgical procedure. My patient had some mild inflammation in her liver related to her chemotherapy treatment. I felt it safest to perform only a liver resection, followed six weeks later by either another three months of chemotherapy or by removal of the colon cancer and then additional chemotherapy. We agreed to make the decision on the most appropriate next treatment step based on her pathology results after she recovered successfully from her liver operation.

Two weeks later I performed an exploratory laparotomy and confirmed she had a tumor in the left side of her colon. It was small and did not obstruct the intestine. I felt no obviously abnormal lymph nodes anywhere near the primary tumor. Intraoperative ultrasound confirmed the presence of five liver tumors, and as happens in 5 or 6 percent of the patients I treat, the ultrasound revealed a single six-millimeter tumor deep in the left lobe of her liver. This tumor was, no doubt, present the entire time, but was simply too small to be detected on the CT imaging. I always warn patients that when I use the direct liver ultrasound I might find a few additional small lesions and that I will deal with them at the time of their operation. I proceeded with removing the entire right lobe of her liver as well as a small portion of the left lobe, to assure a tumor-free resection margin. I finished the operation by performing a microwave ablation of the single small tumor in the left lobe of the liver. The operation went flawlessly, she required no blood transfusions, and she was up, alert and walking the next morning. Her hospital course went smoothly and she was discharged five days later. She was feeling the expected fatigue associated with rapid regeneration of the liver, but was smiling and happy over the results.

But the single small tumor in the left lobe of her liver foreshadowed a problem. I saw this woman a few days after her discharge and she was doing well. I scheduled her to return five weeks later to see me and her medical oncologist with repeat CT imaging to assess her liver regeneration and to discuss the next steps in therapy. When the patient returned for her appointment, one of my surgical residents went in and talked to her first. She came out after a few minutes and reported the patient was feeling well, although she admitted she had a bit of a dry cough and her energy levels, which had been recovering nicely, had waned a bit over the past few days. The resident detected nothing unusual on physical examination, and the patient's surgical scar was healing nicely.

I pulled up the patient's CT scans on the computer and the resident and I gaped at the images. She had dozens of marble-sized tumors in her lungs, and her regenerated left liver was peppered with at least ten golf ball-sized metastases. Unbelievable! I had performed an ultrasound on her liver six weeks earlier and none of these tumors had been evident. An early and aggressive recurrence of cancer after liver resection does not happen very often, but when it does, it is a miserable conversation to have with the patient and family. Eyes initially downcast, I walked dejectedly into her room. The patient knew immediately from my demeanor something was very wrong. I sat and faced her and her husband, looked her directly in the eyes, and I began to describe and explain what I was seeing on her CT scans. She started weeping quietly, but was soon sobbing loudly. Suddenly, from behind me I heard my resident state, "This is too real." I turned to see a stricken expression on the resident's face, her eyes welling with tears. She fled from the room.

I sat with my patient and her husband for another forty minutes and explained further surgical treatment was off the table as an option. Her primary colon cancer was still small and not causing problems. I mentioned we needed to initiate chemotherapy as quickly as possible. I called my medical oncology colleague who was treating her and he kindly dropped what he was doing to come speak with the patient and her husband.

I walked out of the examination room emotionally and physically drained by the conversation and the unfortunate situation this patient faced. She asked impossible-to-answer questions about the probability of seeing her children graduate from college. Her children were still in high school. Given the behavior of her cancer, my medical oncology colleague and I knew we were dealing with a vicious disease running rampant. We hoped to rein it in for at least a while.

After I dropped the bomb of horrible news on the patient and her husband in the examination room, I went searching for my surgical resident. She was nowhere to be found in the clinic. I pulled myself together and went back to work to see some additional patients. About twenty minutes later, my red-eyed resident reappeared. I took her aside into a quiet corner and asked what I could do to assist and support her. She explained that she'd been overcome by grief because her own mother had died the previous year. Ten years prior, her mother had been diagnosed with stage III breast cancer. She had undergone surgical treatment and chemotherapy. For almost a decade, her mother had been cancer-free and living a normal life. Then, unexpectedly, the malignant beast reared its head again and she developed back and leg pain. Scans revealed she had metastatic breast cancer in her liver, lungs, and bones. Ultimately, it also appeared in her brain. She was treated with chemotherapy and radiation therapy but lived less than six months after her diagnosis of metastatic breast cancer. The resident admitted to me she had suppressed much of the emotion related to her mother's death because she had needed to get back to work taking care of surgical patients.

When I was sharing the bad news with my colorectal-cancer patient, however, it had opened a personal Pandora's box for the surgical resident. All of the unresolved feelings regarding her mother's cancer had rushed out and momentarily overwhelmed her. It is a risk all of us face, balancing compassionate and thoughtful care with control of mental turmoil from our own personal situations and our experiences. After we finished the clinic, my resident and I went downstairs to the coffee shop. We talked for half an hour and I encouraged her to speak with me, other faculty, colleagues, or friends about the difficult emotions and to recognize and accept that it was okay to express feelings about her loss. Sometimes a tough facade is fine, even necessary, but not at the expense of true compassion for others and for ourselves.

Things were much worse than we anticipated for my patient who had precipitated the release of the surgical resident's pent-up feelings. The patient's medical oncologist called me the next week to tell me he had admitted her to the hospital. Her liver tumors had grown so rapidly that her liver was beginning to fail. I went to the intensive care unit and visited the patient, her husband, and children. Even the usually tough ICU nurse was crying softly by the end of the conversation. The patient and her husband graciously thanked me for my efforts on her behalf, and she told me how proud she was of her two children. Then she turned to her children and told them she was sorry she was leaving them and to always remember her love and devotion to them.

She died two days later.

Patients, family members, friends, and caregivers treating cancer patients ride a constant emotional roller coaster. There are occasionally thrills as we see patients back in the clinic who are long-term survivors living complete and fulfilling lives. Conversely, there are periods of gloom as we watch patients suffer from toxic treatments while their cancer progresses and ultimately claims their life. Even patients who are doing well years after a cancer diagnosis tell me they get wound up and anxious for a few days before their routine follow-up visit with me or other oncologists involved in their care. Treating patients with cancer is sometimes a viscerally painful, mentally draining, and powerful experience. You can only imagine the profoundly emotional experience for a cancer patient, unless you yourself have been such a patient.

It's not an easy choice, but I choose to feel. I am engaged and involved with my patients, and I'll spend as much time with them as they need. I have many patients whom I follow right up to the time of their death, some of whom I've never operated on. What I have learned is that patients don't want to be abandoned. They want to know that someone will be present and will provide assistance when they have symptoms or fears and need support.

We need to support our own as well. The physicians, nurses, trainees, and all cancer caregivers are devoted to helping patients who are facing a frightening and potentially lethal disease.

We need to remember the emotional toll. We need to take care of all.

30

Be the Dog

"Modesty means admitting the possibility of error, subsuming the self for the good of the whole, remaining open to surprise and the gifts that only failure can bring. There are many ways to practice it. Try taking up golf. Or making your own bagels. Or raising a teenager."

Nancy Gibbs

Modesty: The quality or state of being unassuming in the estimation of one's abilities

My great-grandfather was a reserved, taciturn man. He was in his late seventies and eighties when I was growing up in New Mexico. When he did speak, it was worth listening, because his few words carried impact, perception, or wry humor. I always looked forward to our time together because it represented an opportunity to learn from a master observer who had been born in the late nineteenth century and experienced remarkable progress in the twentieth. He had been a miner, a builder, a hunter, a fly fisherman, an expert in surviving in the high mountains in all

seasons, a self-taught mechanical engineer, and a keen commen-
tator regarding human behavior. His statements on the last were
invariably terse but remarkably insightful.

One day, I walked in to my grandmother's house, where my
great-grandfather sat at the kitchen table with a cup of coffee in
his hand. I asked, "How are you doing today?" He took a sip of
coffee and, never meeting my eyes with his gaze, commented,
"Some days you're the dog; some days you're the tree."

I had learned from previous experience never to ask for an
explanation of his somewhat abstruse remarks. He had told me
once that I should, "Think it through." So this time I sat in a
chair next to him and pondered for a moment. I looked up at him,
and said, "So some days you feel like you're rooted in place and
must endure whatever problems arise and deal with whatever is
dumped on you, while other days you are running happy, free,
and able to leave your mark on the world."

He took another sip of coffee, still staring out the window, and a
small smile played at the corners of his mouth. He gave an almost-
imperceptible, affirmative nod. He then patted me on the arm and
said, "Smart boy."

It was the most emotion I ever saw him express. I was thrilled
to have earned high praise from this occasionally curmudgeonly,
genuinely thoughtful and experienced man. He lived alone in a
small stone house in the Jemez Mountains northwest of Albuquerque. It had a wood-burning stove but no central heating or
air-conditioning. It did have central plumbing that my great-
grandfather had rigged up himself. He had no telephone; if he
wanted to make a call he had to amble down the mountain to the
nearby home of his niece.

In addition to his other skills, my great-grandfather was a master
furniture maker. He created amazing pieces from wood he milled
and shaped himself. He was also able to carve beautiful figures

of animals and birds out of wood or stone. Several of his skillfully cut and polished sculptures are included in the Americana collection at the Smithsonian Institution. I will always display and cherish the wolf he carved for me out of lilac-colored lepidolite. The raw material came from one of the many mine claims throughout northern New Mexico and southern Colorado where my great-grandfather had worked. When he died, I was bequeathed his complete set of hand-carving tools. Sadly, I did not inherit his skill in working with wood and stone, although I am very handy when it comes to carving malignant tumors out of my human patients.

About a month ago, I had a great week. I was the dog. On Monday, I successfully completed a wonderfully symmetrical day by first performing a left hepatectomy for colorectal-cancer metastasis, followed by a right-lobe liver resection in a patient with an intrahepatic cholangiocarcinoma. Both operations went perfectly with minimal blood loss. Both patients were up walking the halls on the surgical ward the night of their operations and asking when a dinner menu would be delivered. On Tuesday I had a splendid day in the clinic. My schedule was full, and I saw several new patients who were candidates for surgical treatment of their malignant disease. The patients and their families were relieved to know I could potentially remove their liver tumors and give them hope of controlling and possibly beating the cancer. As lunchtime approached, the day was interrupted when my physician's assistant tapped me on the shoulder and asked if I was having good day. I replied I was indeed, and I turned around to see the entire clinic staff and all of the surgical residents with a birthday cake. Somebody had leaked the date! I protested (unsuccessfully) that it was false news. They embarrassed me completely by loudly singing "Happy Birthday to You" and I blushingly endured teasing and further birthday songs from my patients for the next several hours. On Wednesday I attended an energizing education session for the residents, and I spent some time individually teaching students and residents about the process of thinking through options and evaluating patients with various malignant diseases. Any chance for me to teach or learn makes for a great day. On Thursday, I completed two more liver operations that went smoothly, and, again, both patients recovered quickly and uneventfully. Friday saw another clinic day following up on patients who were recovering well after liver resections and with no need to drop bad news on anyone. I also met with two patients who were scheduled for operations the next Monday, I answered all questions and went over the details of their procedures to their satisfaction.

Unexpectedly, I received five birthday notes from patients or their family members during the week. The information leak from my staff was worse than I had imagined. One card read, "Hello Dr. Curley. You treated my husband twelve years ago for colon cancer spread to his liver. I am happy to say he is still cancer-free and we have raised our family. Thank you for giving us over a decade more than we were told we would have with him." The five patients—all cancer survivors—were initially told they had "incurable" disease. All had undergone major liver resections and chemotherapy and were enjoying life and family, cancer-free eleven to sixteen years after their surgical treatment.

All in all, a darned good week loping like a carefree dog and leaving a positive mark on the world.

But the following Monday I quickly became the tree. My first patient was scheduled for an operation at 8 a.m., and I had planned to do a straightforward, small-wedge liver resection. All of our detailed, state-of-the-art preoperative imaging studies showed only a single two-centimeter tumor at the edge of the liver. Depending on the type of cancer, I occasionally start some procedures with a diagnostic laparoscopy to view the entire peritoneal cavity, and I ultrasound the liver to make certain there are no additional or small tumors not detected on the preoperative imaging studies. In most patients, I will start with a small mini-laparotomy incision just big enough to allow me to inspect and palpate the organs. I made such an incision in my first patient and upon entering the belly cavity immediately encountered hundreds of tumors smaller than a grain of rice. I biopsied several and while awaiting a frozen-section analysis by our pathologist, I performed an ultrasound of the liver. More shocking news: there were dozens of liver tumors scattered in every portion of the liver, each only three or four millimeters in size. I biopsied one near the surface of the liver and went to the frozen-section room to look through the microscope with the pathologist. All of the tumors were the same type as the one we had already planned to take out. The operation was over because there was no way to remove all of the malignancies.

My resident and I closed the small laparotomy incision. I went out to deliver the grim news to the family. It was not received well. The patient had more than a dozen family members present, and they expressed a full gamut of emotion, from anger to disbelief to sobbing sadness. I waited for approximately an hour after the operation, and once the patient was awake, I repeated the conversation with the patient. Again, it was not well received. How could it be? I felt sad, frustrated, and stuck in place because I had not been able to help the patient.

I started the second operation that day in the same fashion, with a small incision. Thankfully, I found no tumors in the peritoneal cavity. My relief was short lived, however, because once again ultrasound revealed that instead of only two tumors in the right lobe of the liver that could be easily removed surgically, there were dozens of small tumors scattered throughout every segment of the liver. Again, biopsies confirmed diffuse malignant disease throughout the organ. The incision was sutured closed. I took the

seemingly interminable, long, shuffling walk to the surgical waiting area and delivered the unfortunate news. It was not even noon
on Monday and I already felt physically and emotionally drained
and bedraggled.

On Tuesday the clinic started well with a new patient who
was a surgical candidate and follow-up patients with assessments
revealing they were tumor-free. After I delivered the good news,
there were sighs of relief, smiles, and hugs in each room. Then
the roof caved in. A young patient, whom I admire greatly for her
determination and grit, came in for a follow-up visit three years
after I had removed a primary cancer from her liver. This lady had
amazed her medical oncologist and me by running two miles to
and from her weekly chemotherapy sessions before and after her
liver operation. She told us, "I feel like hell, but pushing through
the sickness gives me purpose and hope." She has impressive spirit
and willpower. Her tumor blood marker, which had been normal
for three years, was now elevated. I opened her scan images on a
computer terminal and my heart sank. There were several new
tumors in the hypertrophied liver and numerous enlarged lymph
nodes near the blood vessels in her abdomen. I entered the examination room, and she and her husband knew immediately I was
about to drop bad-news napalm on them. I maintained a calm
and professional facade and quietly explained the findings indicating her cancer had recurred. After I finished describing the
situation, there was uncomfortable silence in the room.

Dumbfounded, she looked into my eyes and said, "How can
this be? I am one who was supposed to beat cancer."

I had no response.

We talked for another fifteen minutes or so, and I called her
medical oncologist to let him know the situation. He was disappointed and deflated, too. He started her on a new chemotherapy
regimen and we will follow closely and see what happens. My

patient had asked me during our clinic visit if she would ever again be a candidate for an operation to remove any remaining cancer. I answered honestly; it was not likely, but with a dramatic response to chemotherapy, I was willing to push the envelope and give her every chance. A true statement for every patient I see. But sadly, far too many patients have cancer my colleagues and I cannot treat with surgery.

When I arrived at my office Wednesday morning I looked at my schedule and I audibly groaned. The day was packed with nine hours of back-to-back meetings and committees. I don't mind administrative duties if something is achieved and progress and decisions are made. But I knew from the list of meetings that that was not going to happen. I girded myself emotionally and sat through a day of verbose entropy. I participated actively, but, as predicted, no tangible success, decisions, or plans were made. I was far more exhausted at day's end than I would have been after a similar day in the operating room. Thankfully, my single complex, six-hour operation on Thursday was successful, and I was pleased to be released from three days of bad karma. Nonetheless, I walked out recognizing the operation was for a cancer with a high propensity to metastasize and leave microscopic deposits of malignancy elsewhere in the body. More treatment will be needed for this patient, and then we will begin the process of nervous watchfulness. It is a tough existence for patients, family, friends, and the medical team. On Friday the clinic was completed uneventfully and with no more bad news to drop on patients. Whew! I met with my research team Friday afternoon and we reviewed several manuscripts and laboratory results. We planned a set of experiments needed to finish projects, knowing a long period of our work was coming to an end. It was time to move on to new ideas and new research to find (hopefully) better treatments for our patients.

As I drove home Friday afternoon I reflected on the previous two weeks. One of the messages I had received from a patient the week of my birthday thanked me for being "the world's greatest doctor" and for being responsive and caring. I appreciated the sentiment, and while comments like this may be great for the ego, they must be kept in some rational and realistic perspective. There is no world's greatest doctor. The world contains lots of great, well-trained, hard-working, caring physicians. There are no Olympics for liver surgeons, oncologists, or other types of medical providers. No gold medals, no world records to beat, no objective measures of who is the best. All of us involved in cancer care should strive to do our best for each patient. It is critically important to have an honest and caring relationship with our patients, but such a goal is not always achieved. The demands, stresses, failures, complications, side effects, and sometimes brutal reality of cancer's effect on patients, caregivers, and clinicians can conspire to produce frustration, angst, disappointment, and burnout.

Too many times, cancer still defeats our attempts, no matter how great a job we do with our multidisciplinary treatments; the high-quality, complex cancer operations; the formulation and delivery of anticancer therapeutics; and the complicated three- and four-dimensional ionizing-radiation planning and delivery. Look at the statistics. Despite remarkable advances in basic science and clinical research over the past four decades, cancer is still the second most common cause of death in Western countries, and it is rapidly closing in on heart disease to become the most common. That is good reason to temper any egocentricity or arrogance among cancer clinicians; we have a painfully obvious high rate of failure. Cancer still wins the battle far too often.

None of us can be the dog all the time.

In 2021 we will mark the fiftieth anniversary of the war on cancer. The war will continue for many years after 2021. I am hopeful and optimistic that we will continue to make progress; continue to advance on the enemy; and through ongoing developments in research and understanding of this nefarious disease, our success rates will be higher and our patients will live longer, productive lives. We must maintain hope, courage, and commitment. I am reminded by my patients every day of the importance of working to sustain these qualities.

I am grateful, and I am blessed to have the privilege of providing care for patients battling cancer. My colleagues and I will fight alongside them and help as we can. And I will offer the same four words to all: "Always happy to help."

ACKNOWLEDGMENTS

I have written many surgical, clinical research, and scientific papers or book chapters during the course of my career. I have also edited a couple of textbooks. This first endeavor into a (hopefully) more readable, wider public audience–style of writing has been enjoyable, educational, and energizing. It has allowed me to honor the humanity, spirit, and journey of the cancer patients described herein and to recognize the highs and lows faced by every cancer patient and those who support them. It has helped me manage some of the emotional distress my colleagues and I face as cancer care providers. I have more people to thank for the gifts and blessings they have bestowed upon me throughout my life than can be listed in this brief section, but first and foremost, I thank all the cancer patients and their families who have entrusted me with their care over the years. I cherish the confidence they have placed in me, and I always respect the determination, endurance, and strength they show as they live and work through the diagnosis and treatment of cancer.

I thank my mother for fostering and supporting my love of reading and investigation. Thank you to my father for teaching me the importance of hard work and the stubborn tenacity needed to overcome obstacles or problems placed before me. I am grateful for my son, Niel, and my daughter Emily. You were and are a constant source of joy and challenge for me—with the exception of the teenage years, which we will not discuss any further. Thank you to their spouses, Chelsea and Jess, for their love and support for my offspring. I am grateful to my two youngest daughters, Sarah and Katherine, because I come home every day to new adventures, wonders, and experiences seen through their eyes. Niel and Chelsea have blessed me with two grandchildren, Everly and Nash, who amaze me with their energy, rapid development, and endearing behaviors. And yes, Everly really did need a four-foot-tall stuffed unicorn for her birthday. You are welcome. It will only get worse; this is how Grandpa rolls.

I am committed to teaching students at all levels of education, and I am fortunate to encounter undergraduate, graduate, medical school, and resident physician trainees on a regular basis. An opportunity to teach is always an opportunity to learn, and I thank them for their insightful and thoughtful questions. I teach to honor all who taught me throughout my educational career. I had the good fortune of having teachers throughout primary and secondary school who recognized that I needed extra work and projects to keep me occupied, and I appreciate all of those who took the time to ply me with additional work and reading materials. Medical school is an arduous experience, but Dr. Cheves Smythe and Dr. Benjy Brooks, in particular, provided critical life lessons about caring for patients and maintaining balance in life. Surgical residency was a six-year marathon, including one year of basic science research, and the residents I trained with were a brilliant and bodacious group. I have the utmost admiration for the surgical faculty who had major impact on my training as a young surgical resident, especially Dr. Raymond Doberneck, Dr. William Sterling, Dr. Dan Smith, and Dr. Sterling Edwards. Advanced surgical oncology training was made more rewarding because of the time spent teaching by Dr. David Hohn,

Dr. Charles Balch, Dr. Mark Roh, Dr. Fred Ames, and Dr. Raphael Pollock. The latter individual is a dear friend whose support and assistance throughout the years has earned my enduring love and esteem.

I appreciate the friendship of some of the incredible surgical oncologists with whom I trained, particularly Dr. Merrick Ross and Dr. Mark Talamonti. I had the very good fortune to serve as the surgical oncology fellowship program director at the University of Texas MD Anderson Cancer Center for nineteen years. I am honored to have worked with spectacular fellows from 1990–2014. In 2014, I was granted the marvelous opportunity to work with medical students and surgical residents at the Baylor College of Medicine. These inquisitive and talented people keep me on my toes and inspire me to achieve excellence in all my endeavors. My colleagues in surgical oncology, the department of surgery, and the Dan L Duncan Comprehensive Cancer Center at Baylor are a remarkable and dedicated group of master clinicians.

I have maintained a translational basic research laboratory throughout my career, and the opportunity to work with college undergraduate and graduate students, postdoctoral fellows, and young faculty has pushed me continuously to find better treatments for patients with malignant disease. Working alongside my colleagues in all disciplines involved in the diagnosis, treatment, and care for patients with cancer has been an integral component in the successful development of state-of-the-art multidisciplinary treatment programs. I appreciate the commitment to excellence embodied by each of you in the care you provide for our patients. The thousands of nurses, physician's assistants, nurse practitioners, other medical practitioners, support staff, and administrative staff involved in care for our patients deserve a prolonged and heartfelt standing ovation. We could not achieve the desired outcomes in our patients without your commitment and assistance.

I thank, in particular, Veronica Smith for sticking with me for many years now and for providing a level of communication and compassion to our patients that is extraordinary.

Finally, this first-time foray into book publishing has been shepherded by my agent, Jan Miller. Her humor and energy, along with very direct evaluation of my work, has been just what this surgeon needed. *Grazie*, Jan! Delysia Aldana and Ivonne Ortega at Dupree Miller have always graciously answered my inane questions and have patiently responded to emails. I am indebted to Becky Nesbitt and Dorothea Halliday, who have assisted in editing this book. Grace Tweedy Johnson readily responds to my inquiries to the publisher, and I am grateful to the editorial director at Center Street, Kate Hartson, for her unwavering support. And finally, to Kristine Ash and Sandra Palacios, a massive thank-you for your assistance in typing the numerous drafts of chapters in this book. My fingers would not have survived unscathed without your assistance.

INDEX

ABOUT THE AUTHOR

Dr. Steven Curley is professor of surgery, chief of surgical oncology, and director of clinical programs in the Dan L Duncan Comprehensive Cancer Center at the Baylor College of Medicine in Houston, Texas. He has been an academic surgical oncologist for almost thirty years. His surgery practice focuses on patients with gastrointestinal malignancies, particularly cancers involving the liver and pancreas. He maintains a translational basic science laboratory directed toward developing, testing, and performing clinical trials on novel devices to treat patients with malignant tumors. His work led to use of thermal ablation techniques to destroy liver tumors that could not otherwise be removed surgically. His research group is working to develop less invasive, less toxic, and more effective treatments for patients with highly lethal malignant diseases such as pancreatic and primary liver cancer. He has been active throughout his career initiating screening programs to diagnose cancer at early, more treatable stages of disease and in improving multidisciplinary treatments for patients with gastrointestinal cancers. He lives in the Houston area with his wife and two youngest daughters. His son and older daughter are successful young professionals. He shares his space with four dogs, six chickens, and a horse.